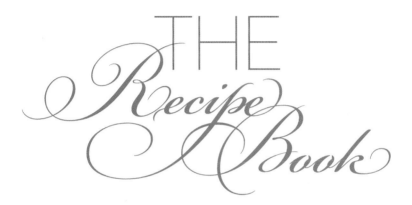

THE Recipe Book

WITH
JEN O'SULLIVAN

The Recipe Book with Jen O'Sullivan

ISBN-13: 978-1720835387
ISBN-10: 1720835381

Printed in the United States of America

November 2018

This book is dedicated to all you oily geeks out there! You know who you are. You can't get enough recipes and are always on the hunt for the latest and greatest. With over 250 recipes for emotions, the mind, the body, children, dogs, personal fragrance, and even infused wine, beer, and coffee, this book will give you fun ways to use your essential oils through rollers, serums, spritzers, diffusing, layering, and even some fun belly button methods. Enjoy the journey and live well!

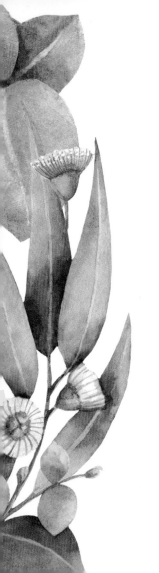

Capture the
Essence of
Life

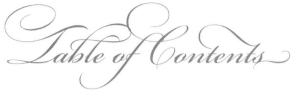

Table of Contents

8 EDUCATIONAL RESOURCES
9 INTRODUCTION
12 BASIC SUPPLY LIST
13 EXPERT ADVICE

Section One
18 *SPOTLIGHT:* White Angelica™
19 EMOTIONAL HEALTH
20 Anger
21 Annoyance
22 Betrayal
23 Bitterness
24 Broken Heart
26 Confidence
27 Courage
28 Emotional Frailty
29 Energy
30 Frustration
31 Gratitude
32 Grief
33 Grounding
34 Happiness

35 Hopelessness
36 Peaceful
37 Peacemaker
38 Security
39 Thanks
49 Unicorn
41 Worry

Section Two
42 *SPOTLIGHT:* Sacred Frankincense™
43 MENTAL HEALTH
44 Aging Gracefully
45 Boredom
46 Calming
47 Confusion
48 Clarity
49 Energy
50 Focus
51 Focus Calming
52 Focus Layering
53 Invigorating

Section Three

54 *SPOTLIGHT:* Ravintsara
55 PHYSICAL HEALTH
56 Appetite
57 Armpit Serums
58 Breast Health
59 Breathing Support
60 Bugs - Summertime
61 Bugs - Outdoors
62 Eye Area Serums
63 Face Serums
64 Hair Serums
66 Head Health
68 Jet Lag
69 Menopause
70 Motion Balance
71 Nose Dryness
72 Nail Beds
73 Oola Balance™
74 Oola Faith™
75 Oola Family™
76 Oola Field™
77 Oola Finance™
78 Oola Fitness™
79 Oola Friends™
80 Oola Fun™
81 Oola Grow™

82 Respiration
83 Scalp Itch
84 Singer Spray
85 Skin Support
86 Sleep - Belly Button
87 Sleep Angel
88 Stinky Feet
89 Tender Tendons
90 Withdrawal Protocol

Section Four

92 *SPOTLIGHT:* Melaleuca
93 CHILDREN & DOGS
94 Baby Bottom Softening
95 Bed Wetting
96 Bugs - School-age Critters
97 Homework Motivation
98 Teasing
99 Temperature
100 School Focus
101 Sleeping Baby
102 Dog - Furniture Care
103 Dog - Lawn Care
104 Dog - Outdoor Spray
105 Dog - Puppy Re-homing
106 Dog - Stink
107 Dog - Stress

Section Five
108 *SPOTLIGHT:* Jasmine
109 FRAGRANCE
110 Accomplished
111 Awakened
112 Balanced
113 Burly Man
114 Calmed
115 Chai Tea
116 Crystal
117 Courageous
118 Decompresser
119 Dreamy
120 Freedom Fresh
121 Fresh Air
122 Freshly Bright
123 Grateful
124 Grounded
125 Happy Place
126 Ice Cream Delight
127 Inspire
128 Island Dreams
130 Manpower
131 Peace
132 Pumpkin Pie
133 Romantical Nights

134 Seashore Breeze
135 Simplify
136 Spirit Lifter
137 Strength
138 Uplift
139 Worry Free

Section Six
140 *SPOTLIGHT:* Jade Lemon™
141 INFUSED BEVERAGE
142 Infused Beer
143 Infused Champagne
144 Infused Coffee
145 Infused Lemonade
146 Infused NingXia Red®
147 Infused Shakes
148 Infused Water
149 Infused Wine

BONUS RECIPES
150 Infused Chocolate
151 One Hundred Gifts

153 FINAL THOUGHTS
156 RESOURCES

EDUCATIONAL RESOURCES

Jen's Main Educational Group:
www.Facebook.com/groups/TheHumanBody

Shareable Facebook Content & Recipes:
www.Facebook.com/JenOSullivanAuthor

Instagram: @JenAuthor

YouTube: www.JensTips.com

Printed Resources: www.31oils.com

Apps: "The EO Bar" and "Live Well with Young Living"

Vitality Book Educational Video Series:
www.Facebook.com/groups/VitalityBook

Free 15 day eCourse: www.31oils.com/oils101

BOOKS:
The Essential Oil Truth: The Facts Without the Hype
French Aromatherapy: Essential Oil Recipes and Usage Guide
Vitality: The Young Living Lifestyle
Essential Oil Make & Takes
Live Well (the PSK educational mini book)
The Recipe Book with Jen O'Sullivan
Essentially Driven, Young Living Essential Oils Business Handbook

INTRODUCTION

Essential oil users all over the world are on an endless mission to find just the right blend, just the right method, and just the right recipe for their needs. The thrill and excitement that follows with triumph, directly after finding a new recipe that gives great results, is something that propels us further on the journey of natural health solutions.

We find ourselves becoming more and more brave and bold with our usage; we enjoy sharing our triumphs with others; we bask in the glory of doing it ourselves! My hat is off to you, my friend, so keep up the good work! This book is for the seeker. It is for the one who loves the endless possibilities when it comes to natural solutions for health and wellness.

Welcome! My name is Jen O'Sullivan. I am the author of many best-selling aromatherapy books on Amazon and am known for my copious and tireless efforts to educate the world on essential oil use through my multiple free resources online via Facebook, Instagram, and YouTube (see resources to the left). I've been using essential oils since 2007 and have studied whole-body health, wellness, and nutrition since that time to help me not only find a more vitality-filled life, but to teach others how they may obtain health, balance, and freedom too.

I have studied French Aromatherapy and have a certificate in French Medicinal Aromatics through the New York School for Aromatic Studies under the tutelage of Jade Shutes and Cathy Skipper. In the words of long-time oiler, Shannon Hudson, "Jen O'Sullivan believes that getting to the root of the problem is vital to full health and restoration and utilizes a whole-body system approach of care with her students."

In my past professional life, I was a commercial and celebrity photographer, as well as a professor at my alma mater, Art Center College of Design in Pasadena, California. One thing I learned in art school is that you need to know the rules before you break the rules. The same is true with essential oil recipe making.

As one of the largest online essential oil educators, I find there is a vast array of users with varying opinions and methods. I applaud them all as long as they are safe. Essential oils are God's gift to us for our benefit. They are a tremendous blessing!

My goal is to teach you logical methods from the French Aromatherapy school of use. This means you will learn, in some recipes, how to apply neat, without a carrier oil, and in others, how to safely use some oils internally as flavoring. For those of you who want recipes for therapeutic internal use, such as capsules, see my book "French Aromatherapy". In this recipe book, you will even find that I teach specific ways to use oils as well as synergize oils that you may have not learned in the past, even if you are a seasoned user!

I encourage you to be teachable. It has served me well in the past four decades to love the art of learning and always continue to desire growth. No one person knows everything; we do the best we can with what we know and where we are. One step at a time is all it takes to move forward, so keep moving forward, friend!

On the next pages are my simple expert tips that you may want to consider as you formulate your own recipes. As you move through the rest of this recipe book, remember to have fun, share with friends, and enjoy the journey!

~ Jen O'Sullivan

PS: As you make the recipes in this book and come up with your own, I encourage you to use the hashtag #myEOcreation so we can all learn and enjoy these little gems together!

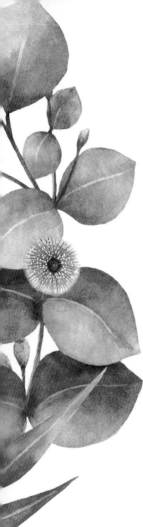

BASIC SUPPLY LIST

Young Living Essential Oils®

For product links see www.31oils.com/supplies

Containers:
- 5mL and 15mL cleaned Young Living® amber bottles
- 15mL dropper tops
- AromaGlide™ Metal roller fitments (from Young Living®)
- 2 oz., 4 oz., and 8 oz. amber or cobalt glass spray bottles

Carrier oils:
- V-6™ Vegetable Oil Complex (from Young Living®)
- Fractionated Coconut
- Grapeseed
- Jamaican Black Castor
- Jojoba
- Mustard Seed
- Neem
- Rosehip Seed
- Sweet Almond

Miscellaneous:
- Alkaline water
- Distilled water
- Pink Himalayan Sea Salt
- Toothpicks
- Vanilla absolute
- Vinegar

EXPERT ADVICE

PRO TIP:

Keep all your essential oils in an upright position.

REASON:

Essential oils are volatile. When they are on their sides, in a drawer or in your purse, they will evaporate slowly or quickly depending on how well you close your lids.

PRO TIP:

Keep all your essential oils caps taut not tight.

REASON:

Under-tightening an essential oil bottle cap will cause the oils to evaporate, but over-tightening them will cause the cap to crack and once that happens, the oils will also evaporate. Keep them just snug enough to not move.

PRO TIP:

Try to not touch the orifice reducer on the essential oil bottle.

REASON:

Any debris, in the form of skin cells and body oils mixed with dust particles and other possible fragments from your fingers, will end up in your oils and will contaminate them in the form of oxidative stress. The more you touch the orifice reducer, the more oxidative stress you add to your oils. They will lower in frequency and therapeutic value. Some essential oils, when touched too often over a long period of time, will become harsh on your skin with signs presenting as a red area or rash-type dermal response. When using roll-ons, try to use them up completel within 6 months or make sure your skin is clean before applying.

PRO TIP:

Create very small batches that will be used within a month or so.

REASON:

Creating small batches can help when determining if you like the desirec aroma and effect of a recipe. It will eliminate the sadness and frustration of losing essential oils when a recipe goes awry. Making a smaller batch to use within one month of creation helps keep your creation fresh. Larger batches that are used over the course of several months have a higher potential of going rancid.

PRO TIP:

Swirl your blends, don't shake them.

REASON:

Shaking essential oils oxygenates them. The more you shake, the more oxygen enters into the molecular structure of the essential oil, causing it to go bad. Unadulterated distilled essential oils do not expire. Cold-pressed essential oils, such as citrus oils, expire in 6-12 months depending on how they are stored. Shaking an essential oil blend right at the beginning of creation is fine, but if it is possible to swirl, do so.

PRO TIP:

Refrigerate your carrier oils.

REASON:

Carrier oils such as grapeseed and coconut have a shelf life of around 6 months. When stored in the refrigerator, they will last for up to 12 months. To know if your carrier oil has gone rancid, smell it. Most cold-pressed, organic, raw, pure carrier oils have very mild to no aroma. Rancid carrier oil smells musty. If your rollerball creation smells "off" to you, throw it away. Using rancid carrier oil is the cause of skin reactions usually in the form of redness and rash. If you create lots of rollerballs that contain more than 50% ratio carrier oil, consider keeping them in your refrigerator.

PRO TIP:

Cold-water vs. nebulizing diffusers

REASON:

You will find all the diffuser recipes in this book labeled as "Cold-water diffuser" recipes. In traditional aromatherapy circles, the term aromatherapy through use of a diffuser usually means a nebulizer and not a cold-water diffuser. When you see directions to only diffuse for 10-20 minutes, it is because it is referencing a nebulizer, such as the Young Living® AromaLux™ diffuser. This book is full of recipes that are meant to be used with a cold-water diffuser and not a nebulizer. There are other types of "diffusers" on the market that use heat. I do not ever recommend the use of heat burners or steamers with therapeutic grade essential oils. Using heat causes the molecules to separate more rapidly and the lighter molecules will burn off first, leaving a fractionated essential oil experience that is not beneficial.

PRO TIP:

Clean your diffuser at least once a week.

REASON:

The instructions tell us to clean it after each use. If that is you, I applaud you. However, most of us forget and can go months without cleaning it, if ever. Make it a ritual to clean your diffuser every Sunday night, or choose a day that works for you so you do not forget.

PRO TIP:

Create a synergy of your desired blend before using it.

REASON:

When you first started oiling, you most likely learned to drip oils from the bottle one at a time into the water of your diffuser. You also most likely learned to fill your roller bottle up with carrier oil first and then add the various essential oils to the bottle. Both of these methods are not the best method because the essential oils will not fully blend. Water and essential oils do not blend or emulsify. Carrier oils and essential oils also do not blend or emulsify.

When you drip single essential oils one at a time into either water or carrier oil, some of the essential oil molecules get encapsulated by the water or carrier oil. Some essential oils will combine and synergize, but most will not. It is best to create a synergy of the blend you desire to use first in a clean bottle.

How to create a synergy: Add all essential oils to the bottle, swirl to blend. Allow the blend to sit for 24 hours to allow all essential oils to fully synergize together. Essential oils are VOCs (Volatile Organic Compounds) and they will synergize if left alone because it is in their nature to do so. Once they are synergized, you may then add the desired amount of drops to a cold-water diffuser, serum, or rollerball.

17

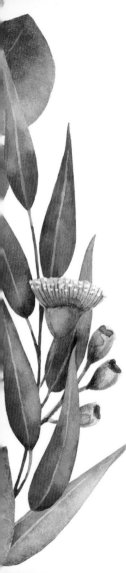

SPOTLIGHT ON WHITE ANGELICA™

White Angelica™ is one of the most popular essential oils for emotional support. We rub it on our chest to help guard against other's negativity. Angelica is an oil that is sometimes confused with White Angelica™. There is more to these two oils than just their names. They are vastly different, but like all essential oils, there are always similarities. When you see a recipe call for one of these oils, you should not use the other as a substitute if you are out, because they don't work the same. Both are used for energy balance but from different ends of the spectrum. Here's a break down of some of their major differences.

ANGELICA
- A single species essential oil from the roots of the Apiaceae family.
- Very high in cleansing Monoterpenes.
- Helps release your own negative energy.

WHITE ANGELICA™
- A blend of Melissa, Northern Lights Black Spruce™, Sacred Sandalwood™, Myrrh, Hyssop, Rose, Geranium, Bergamot, Ylang Ylang, and Coriander with a small amount of Sweet Almond Oil.
- There is no Angelica in White Angelica™.
- High in calming Sesquiterpenes.
- Helps guard against other people's negative energy.

EMOTIONAL HEALTH

Recipes

Anger

Supports: Feelings of emotional stability and calming

Type: Topical Rollerball

Ingredients:
- 10 drops Bergamot
- 10 drops Tangerine
- 5 drops Roman Chamomile
- Carrier oil

Directions: Combine all essential oils to create a synergy in a 5mL rollerball. Swirl to blend, and allow to synergize for 24 hours. Top off with V-6™ carrier oil or carrier of your choosing. Rub on bottom of feet, wrists, and back of neck.

Annoyance

Supports: Feelings of emotionally calm nerves

Type: Topical Rollerball

Ingredients:
- 10 drops Copaiba
- 8 drops Royal Hawaiian Sandalwood™
- 3 drops Coriander
- 3 drops Blue Tansy
- 1 drop Geranium
- Carrier oil

Directions: Combine all essential oils to create a synergy in a 5mL rollerball. Swirl to blend, and allow to synergize for 24 hours. Top off with V-6™ carrier oil or carrier of your choosing. Rub on bottom of feet, wrists, and back of neck as needed.

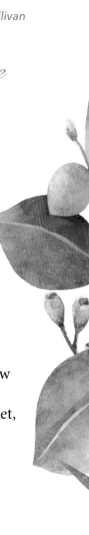

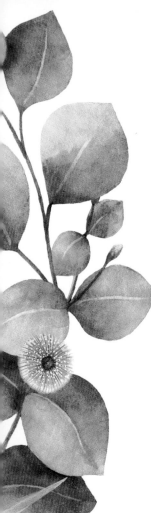

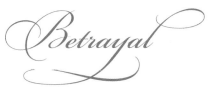

Betrayal

Supports: Feelings of calm and freedom

Type: Cold-water Diffuser Blend

Ingredients:

Recipe #1
- 4 drops Forgiveness™
- 3 drops Orange
- 2 drops Vetiver
- 2 drops Cedarwood

Recipe #2
- 4 drops Ylang Ylang
- 2 drops Melissa
- 2 drops Peppermint

Directions: Add oils to your cold-water diffuser and diffuse for 2-4 hours to help release emotions.

NOTE: You may convert these recipes to a 5mL rollerball. Double the recipe and combine all essential oils into a 5mL rollerball bottle, swirl to blend, and let synergize for 24 hours before topping off with V-6™ or Fractionated Coconut carrier oil. Apply on wrists and back of neck as needed.

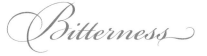

Bitterness

Supports: Feelings of emotional acceptance and resolve

Type: Layering

Ingredients:

Recipe #1:
- 1 drop Copaiba
- 1 drop Joy®
- 1 drop Melissa
- 1 drop Sacred Frankincense™
- Carrier oil

Recipe #2:
- 1 drop Copaiba
- 1 drop Geranium
- 1 drop Orange
- 1 drop Peppermint
- Carrier oil

Directions: Rub the oils one at a time over your heart in a clockwise rotation. If you have sensitive skin, start by rubbing 3 drops of carrier oil, such as V-6™ or Grapeseed. Start with the first oil by dripping it on your chest plate area and rubbing it for 30 seconds. Continue this method with each oil in the above order.

Broken Heart

Supports: Emotional trauma due to loss of love or loss of life

Type: Layering Method (Rollerball on next page)

Ingredients:
- 1 drop Copaiba
- 1 drop Helichrysum
- 1 drop Lavender
- 1 drop Bergamot
- 1 drop Rose
- Carrier oil

Directions: For the first area, start with the first essential oil by rubbing it directly over your heart in a clockwise motion for 30 seconds, then rub the remainder down the inside of your left arm from your underarm to your wrist and down to your pinky finger.

For the second area, add another drop of the same oil to your palm. Rub your hands together gently in a clockwise motion then place both palms directly onto the balls of each foot directly behind your big toes. Place your right hand on your left foot and your left hand on your right foot. Hold that position for 30 seconds, then cup your hands over your nose and breathe in slowly and deeply for three rounds. Move to the next essential oil in the recipe ingredient list and repeat the entire process for both area one and two. Do this for each essential oil. When you are finished you may apply carrier oil if needed. Take a final deep breath from your hands and then rub the remainder of the oils on the back of your neck.

Broken Heart Rollerball Recipe

Ingredients:
- 8 drops Lavender
- 5 drops Copaiba
- 5 drops Helichrysum
- 4 drop Bergamot
- 2 drops Rose (Do not substitute. Leave out if you don't have it.)
- Carrier oil

Directions: Add all essential oils to a 5mL bottle with a metal roller fitment. Swirl to blend, and allow to synergize for 24 hours. Top off with carrier oil of your choice. Rub it on your heart and down your left inner arm to your pinky finger. Rub some onto your palms and inhale deeply for three rounds. Rub the remainder from your palms on the back of your neck.

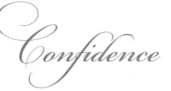

Confidence

Supports: Feelings of focus and grounding

Type: Topical Rollerball

Ingredients:
Recipe #1:
- 15 drops Northern Lights Black Spruce™
- 10 drops Bergamot
- 5 drops Frankincense
- Carrier oil

Recipe #2:
- 10 drops Cedarwood
- 10 drops Grapefruit
- 8 drops Cardamom
- Carrier oil

Directions: Combine all essential oils into a 5mL rollerball bottle, swirl to blend, and let synergize for 24 hours before topping off with V-6™ or Fractionated Coconut carrier oil. Apply on wrists, back of neck, and big toes 2-4 times per day or as needed.

26

Courage

Supports: Feelings of courage, stability, and grounding

Type: Layering

Ingredients:
- 1 drop Copaiba
- 1 drop Valor®
- 1 drop Cypress
- 1 drop Northern Lights Black Spruce™
- Carrier oil

Directions: Rub the oils one at a time over your heart in a clockwise rotation. If you have sensitive skin, start by rubbing 3 drops of carrier oil, such as V-6™ or Grapeseed. Start with the first oil by dripping it on your chest and rubbing it for 30 seconds then rub your hand on the back of your neck for an additional 15 seconds. Continue this method with each oil in the above order. Finish with one drop of carrier oil rubbed on your chest and then on the back of your neck.

Emotional Frailty

Supports: To uplift your spirits during the day and help you drift off to a care-free sleep.

Type: Topical Rollerball

Ingredients:
- 10 drops Valor®
- 5 drops Frankincense
- 3 drops Angelica
- 1 drop Geranium

Directions: Add all essential oils to a 5mL bottle with a metal roller fitment. Swirl to blend, and allow to synergize for 24 hours. Top off with V-6™, Fractionated Coconut oil, or carrier oil of your choice. Apply over your heart and down your inner left arm from your under arm to your palm and pinky finger. Apply to the back of your neck up to your hairline.

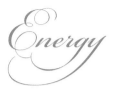

Energy

Supports: Feelings of uplifted emotions

Type: Topical Rollerball

Ingredients:
- 15 drops Orange
- 10 drops Peppermint
- 5 drops Lemon Myrtle
- Carrier oil

Directions: Combine all essential oils into a 5mL rollerball bottle, swirl to blend, and let synergize for 24 hours before topping off with V-6™ or Fractionated Coconut carrier oil. Apply on wrists, back of neck, and chest 2-4 times per day or as needed. Caution when used on skin that may be exposed to the sun.

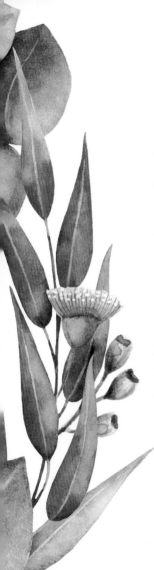

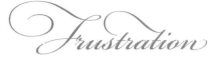

Frustration

Supports: Healthy feelings during frustrating times

Type: Topical Rollerball

Ingredients:
- 20 drops Ylang Ylang
- 10 drops Vetiver
- 2 drops Rose
- Carrier oil

Directions: Combine all essential oils into a 5mL rollerball bottle, swirl to blend, and let synergize for 24 hours before topping off with V-6™ or Fractionated Coconut carrier oil. Apply on wrists, back of neck, and over heart 2-4 times per day or as needed.

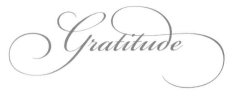

Supports: Feelings of thankfulness

Type: Cold-water Diffuser Blend

Ingredients:

Recipe #1:
- 3 drops Lemon
- 2 drops Geranium
- 2 drops Wintergreen
- 2 drops Spearmint

Recipe #2:
- 3 drops Gratitude™
- 2 drops Tangerine
- 2 drops Peppermint

Directions: Add oils to your cold-water diffuser and diffuse for 2-4 hours.

NOTE: You may convert this recipe to a 5mL rollerball. Combine all essential oils into a 5mL rollerball bottle, swirl to blend, and let synergize for 24 hours before topping off with V-6™ or Fractionated Coconut carrier oil. Apply on wrists, back of neck, and over heart as needed.

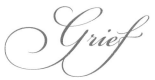

Supports: Comforting feelings during times of loss

Type: Cold-water Diffuser Blend

Ingredients:

Recipe #1:
- 5 drops Bergamot
- 3 drops Frankincense
- 2 drops Vetiver

Recipe #2
- 4 drops Gentle Baby™
- 2 drops Juniper
- 1 drop Sacred Mountain™

Recipe #3
- 4 drops Joy®
- 2 drops Clary Sage
- 2 drops Orange

Recipe #4
- 4 drops Hope™
- 3 drops Tangerine
- 2 drops Hong Kuai

Directions: Add oils to your cold-water diffuser and diffuse for 2-4 hours.

NOTE: You may convert these recipes to a 5mL rollerball. Combine all essential oils into a 5mL rollerball bottle, swirl to blend, and let synergize for 24 hours before topping off with V-6™ or Fractionated Coconut carrier oil. Apply on wrists, back of neck, and over heart 2-4 times per day or as needed.

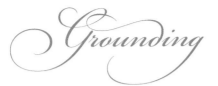

Grounding

Supports: Feelings of being well-grounded and balanced

Type: Topical Rollerball

Ingredients:

Recipe #1:
- 20 drops Northern Lights Black Spruce™
- 10 drops Frankincense
- 10 drops Lavender
- Carrier oil

Recipe #2:
- 15 drops Cypress
- 8 drops Vetiver
- 5 drops Sacred Sandalwood™
- 5 drops Blue Tansy
- 2 drops Pine
- Carrier oil

Directions: Combine all essential oils into a 5mL rollerball bottle, swirl to blend, and let synergize for 24 hours before topping off with V-6™ or Fractionated Coconut carrier oil. Apply on wrists, back of neck, and big toes 2-4 times per day or as needed.

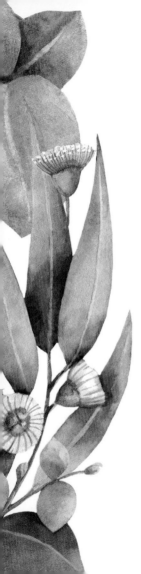

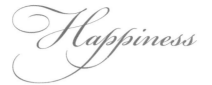

Happiness

Supports: Feelings of happiness

Type: Cold-water Diffuser Blend

Ingredients:
- 4 drops Grapefruit
- 2 drops Lemon
- 2 drops Orange
- 2 drops Peppermint

Directions: Add oils to your cold-water diffuser and diffuse for 2-4 hours.

NOTE: You may convert this recipe to a 5mL rollerball. Double the recipe and combine all essential oils into a 5mL rollerball bottle, swirl to blend, and let synergize for 24 hours before topping off with V-6™ or Fractionated Coconut carrier oil. Apply on wrists, back of neck, and over heart as needed. Do not apply to sun-exposed skin.

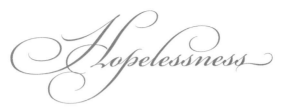

Supports: Feelings of hope

Type: Topical Rollerball

Ingredients:

Recipe #1:
- 10 drops Hope™
- 10 drops Sacred Frankincense™
- 4 drops Lime
- Carrier oil

Recipe #2:
- 15 drops Juniper
- 10 drops Rosemary
- 5 drops Blue Tansy
- Carrier oil

Directions: Combine all essential oils into a 5mL rollerball bottle, swirl to blend, and let synergize for 24 hours before topping off with V-6™ or Fractionated Coconut carrier oil. Apply on wrists, back of neck, and chest 2-4 times per day or as needed.

Peaceful

Supports: Feelings of peace and gratitude

Type: Cold-water Diffuser Blend

Ingredients:
- 4 drops Peace & Calming®
- 3 drops Royal Hawaiian Sandalwood™

Directions: Add oils to your cold-water diffuser and diffuse for 2-4 hours.

NOTE: You may convert this recipe to a 5mL rollerball. Double or triple the recipe and combine all essential oils into a 5mL rollerball bottle, swirl to blend, and let synergize for 24 hours before topping off with V-6™ or Fractionated Coconut carrier oil. Apply on wrists, back of neck, and over heart 2-4 times per day or as needed.

Peacemaker

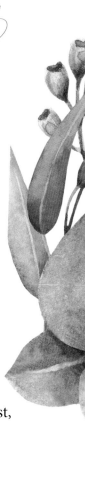

Supports: Feelings of love and unity

Type: Topical Rollerball

Ingredients:
- 10 drops Tangerine
- 8 drops Patchouli
- 5 drops Orange
- 3 drops Ylang Ylang
- Carrier oil

Directions: Combine all essential oils into a 5mL rollerball bottle, swirl to blend, and let synergize for 24 hours before topping off with V-6™ or Fractionated Coconut carrier oil. Apply on wrists, back of neck, chest, and big toes 2-4 times per day or as needed.

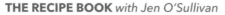

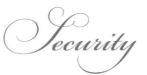

Supports: Feelings of emotional safety and grounding

Type: Topical Rollerball

Ingredients:

Recipe #1:
- 12 drops Gentle Baby™
- 4 drops Orange

Recipe #2
- 8 drops Myrrh
- 8 drops Sacred Sandalwood™
- 4 drops Palo Santo

Recipe #3
- 12 drops White Angelic
- 4 drops Palo Santo
- 4 drops Hong Kuai

Directions: Combine all essential oils into a 5mL rollerball bottle, swirl to blend, and let synergize for 24 hours before topping off with V-6™ or Fractionated Coconut carrier oil. Apply on wrists, back of neck, and over heart 2-4 times per day or as needed.

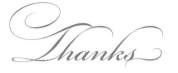

Supports: Feelings of gratitude and balance

Type: Cold-water Diffuser Blend

Ingredients:

Recipe #1:
- 4 drops Tangerine
- 3 drops Gratitude™

Recipe #2:
- 4 drops Orange
- 2 drops Jade Lemon
- 2 drops Nutmeg

Recipe #3:
- 3 drops Kunzea
- 3 drops Sacred Sandalwood™
- 1 drop Jasmine

Recipe #4:
- 6 drops Stress Away™
- 3 drops Lemon Myrtle

Directions: Add oils to your cold-water diffuser and diffuse for 2-4 hours.

NOTE: You may convert these recipes to a 5mL rollerball. Triple the recipe and combine all essential oils from one recipe into a 5mL rollerball bottle, swirl to blend, and let synergize for 24 hours before topping off with V-6™ or Fractionated Coconut carrier oil. Apply on wrists, back of neck, and over heart as needed.

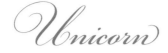

Supports: Healthful feelings of ultra-calm and grounding

Type: Topical Rollerball

Ingredients:
- 5 drops Northern Lights Black Spruce™
- 5 drops Sacred Frankincense™
- 5 drops Sacred Sandalwood™
- 5 drops Roman Chamomile
- 5 drops Copaiba
- 5 drops Vetiver
- 5 drops Cedarwood
- 5 drops Lavender
- 5 drops Blue Tansy
- Carrier oil

Directions: Combine all essential oils into a 5mL rollerball bottle, swirl to blend, and let synergize for 24 hours before topping off with V-6™ or Fractionated Coconut carrier oil. Apply on wrists, back of neck, top of head, and on big toes 2-4 times per day or as needed.

Worry

Supports: Feelings of acceptance and freedom

Type: Layering Method

Ingredients:
- 1 drop Copaiba
- 1 drop Release™
- 2 drops Bergamot
- 1 drop Joy®
- 1 drop Peppermint
- Carrier oil

Directions: Rub the oils one at a time on your left underarm, from your underarm crease down to your elbow. If you have sensitive skin, start by rubbing 2 drops of carrier oil, such as V-6™ or Grapeseed. Start with the first oil and drip it into your right palm, then rub it in small clockwise circular motions from your underarm to your elbow. Continue this method with each oil in the above order, finishing off with a little carrier oil. Cup hands over nose and breathe deeply.

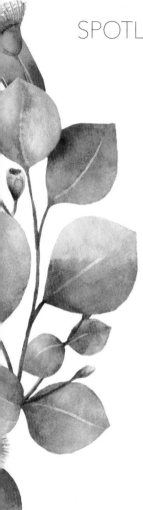

SPOTLIGHT ON SACRED FRANKINCENSE™

Not all Frankincense (from the genus *Boswellia*) essential oils are the same. There over 30 species of *Boswellia*, such as *Boswellia carterii*, *Boswellia frereana*, *Boswellia serrata*, and *Boswellia papyrifera* to name a few. One specific essential oil, called Sacred Frankincense™ (*Boswellia sacra*), is only carried by Young Living®. No company carries Young Living's® true Sacred Frankincense™, but you will see some companies label a version of *Boswellia sacra* as Sacred Frankincense, when it is actually *Boswellia frereana*. In fact, some carry a trio or quad of Frankincense oils, and some even label it as just Frankincense hoping consumers will not notice it is a blend and not a single species! A quick peek at a competitor's website and you will note that their Frankincense is labeled under "Single Oils" yet the ingredients list "Resin from *Boswellia carterii, sacra, papyrifera,* and *frereana*." That is four different species altogether and should not be labeled as a single species.

When you see a recipe in this book that calls for Sacred Frankincense™ and you only have Frankincense, you should not substitute the oils. They are different and do different things for us. It is fun to start seeing how they differ. Generally, Frankincense (*Boswellia carterii*) is the one to use for your skin and for calming, while Sacred Frankincense™ should be used for greater mental clarity and a heightened spiritual awareness. Take a look at their differences below.

MONOTERPENES:

Alpha-Pinenes
Very bioavailable and rapidly metabolizes. Considered a cleansing molecule.
- Sacred Frankincense™ (*Boswellia sacra*) 53-90%
- Frankincense (*Boswellia carterii*) 30-65%

L-Limonene: (chiral or mirror image to D-Limonene)
Skin smoothing support.
- Frankincense (*Boswellia carterii*) 8-20%
- Sacred Frankincense™ (*Boswellia sacra*) 2-7.5 %

SESQUITERPENES: Beta-Caryophyllene

Calming molecules and good for skin.
- Only found in Frankincense (*Boswellia carterii*) 1-5%

SECTION TWO

MENTAL HEALTH

Recipes

Aging Gracefully

Supports: Feelings of confidence and clarity

Type: Topical Rollerball

Ingredients:
- 20 drops Sacred Frankincense™
- 20 drops Helichrysum
- 10 drops Frankincense
- 10 drops Royal Hawaiian Sandalwood™
- 5 drops Rosemary
- Carrier oil

Directions: Combine all essential oils to create a synergy in a 5mL rollerball and swirl bottle to mix well. It is suggested to let sit for 24 hours to fully synergize and then top off with V-6™ carrier oil or carrier of your choosing. Roll on wrists, back of neck, and over chest area. May be used on the back of your hands as well. Allow this aroma to infuse your mind and body with feelings of youthfulness.

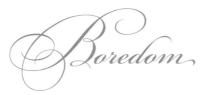

Boredom

Supports: Feelings of motivation and energy

Type: Cold-water Diffuser Blend

Ingredients:

Recipe #1
- 2 drops Motivation™
- 3 drops Tangerine
- 3 drops Wintergreen

Recipe #2
- 5 drops PanAway®
- 3 drops Orange
- 1 drop Rosemary

Directions: Add oils to your cold-water diffuser and diffuse for 2-4 hours.

NOTE: You may convert these recipes to a 5mL rollerball. Double the recipe and combine all essential oils into a 5mL rollerball bottle, swirl to blend, and let synergize for 24 hours before topping off with V-6™ or Fractionated Coconut carrier oil. Apply on wrists and back of neck 2-4 times per day or as needed.

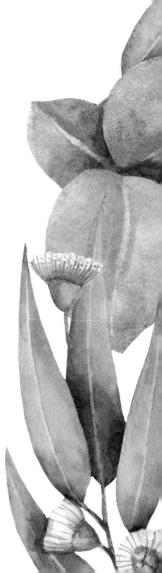

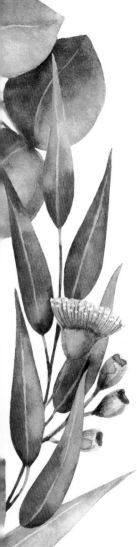

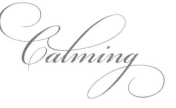

Calming

Supports: General relaxation and calming

Type: Topical Rollerball

Ingredients:
- 15 drops Sacred Frankincense™
- 10 drops Sacred Sandalwood™
- 5 drops Roman Chamomile
- 5 drops Copaiba
- Carrier oil

Directions: Combine all essential oils into a 5mL rollerball bottle, swirl to blend, and let synergize for 24 hours before topping off with V-6™ or Fractionated Coconut carrier oil. Apply on wrists, back of neck, front of neck, and down the sternum 2-4 times per day or as needed.

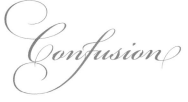

Supports: Clarity of mind

Type: Cold-water Diffuser Blend

Ingredients:

Recipe #1:
- 5 drops Clarity™
- 4 drops Copaiba
- 3 drops Lime

Recipe #2:
- 5 drops Dragon Time™
- 5 drops Copaiba
- 2 drops Spearmint

Recipe #3:
- 4 drops Rosemary
- 3 drops PanAway®
- 3 drops Lemon

Recipe #4:
- 5 drops Peppermint
- 3 drops Melissa
- 2 drops Frankincense

Directions: Add oils to your cold-water diffuser and diffuse for 2-4 hours.

NOTE: You may convert this recipe to a 5mL rollerball. Double the recipe and combine all essential oils into a 5mL rollerball bottle, swirl to blend, and let synergize for 24 hours before topping off with V-6™ or Fractionated Coconut carrier oil. Apply to wrists and back of neck 2-4 times per day or as needed.

Supports: Mental clarity

Type: Layering

Ingredients:

Recipe #1:
- 1 drop Copaiba
- 1 drop Clarity™
- 1 drop Stress Away™

Recipe #2:
- 1 drop Copaiba
- 1 drop Dragon Time™
- 1 drop Rosemary

Recipe #3:
- 1 drop Valor®
- 1 drop Spearmint
- 1 drop Peppermint

Recipe #4:
- 1 drop Copaiba
- 1 drop Rosemary
- 1 drop Peppermint

Directions: Apply each oil one at a time directly to the back of the neck. After each single oil application, cup your application hand over your nose, close your eyes, and breathe in deeply, then move onto the next oil in the recipe. Finish by breathing in the aroma from your application hand 3 full breaths.

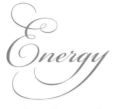

Supports: Feelings of heightened and stimulated awareness

Type: Cold-water Diffuser Blend

Ingredients:
Recipe #1:
- 3 drops Peppermint
- 3 drops Orange

Recipe #2:
- 4 drops En-R-Gee™
- 2 drops Peppermint

Recipe #3
- 5 drops Bergamot
- 2 drops Black Pepper
- 2 drops Nutmeg

Directions: Add oils to your cold-water diffuser and diffuse for 2-4 hours.

NOTE: You may convert these recipes to a 5mL rollerball. Double the recipe and combine all essential oils into a 5mL rollerball bottle, swirl to blend, and let synergize for 24 hours before topping off with V-6™ or Fractionated Coconut carrier oil. Apply on wrists and over heart as needed.

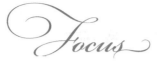

Focus

Supports: Mental clarity during work and study times

Type: Cold-water Diffuser Blend

Ingredients:

Recipe #1:
- 2 drops Frankincense
- 2 drops Cedarwood
- 2 drops Vetiver

Recipe #2:
- 3 drops Northern Lights Black Spruce™
- 3 drops Lavender
- 2 drops Copaiba
- 2 drops Lime

Directions:

Add to a cold-water diffuser and diffuse for 2-4 hours.

NOTE: You may convert these recipes to a 5mL rollerball. Triple the recipe and combine all essential oils into a 5mL rollerball bottle, swirl to blend, and let synergize for 24 hours before topping off with V-6™ or Fractionated Coconut carrier oil. Apply on wrists and back of neck as needed.

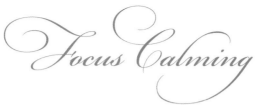

Focus Calming

Supports: Settled and balanced mental clarity

Type: Topical Rollerball

Ingredients:

Recipe #1:
- 15 drops Lime
- 10 drops Cedarwood
- 10 drops Lavender
- 5 drops Sacred Sandalwood™
- 5 drops Copaiba

Recipe #2:
- 10 drops Brain Power™
- 10 drops Copaiba
- 10 drops Sacred Frankincense™

Recipe #3
- 10 drops Royal Hawaiian Sandalwood™
- 5 drops Blue Cypress
- 5 drops Frankincense

Directions: Combine all essential oils into a 5mL rollerball bottle, swirl to blend, and let synergize for 24 hours before topping off with V-6™ or Fractionated Coconut carrier oil. Apply on wrists, back of neck, and across forehead 2-4 times per day or as needed.

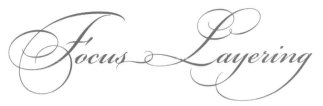

Supports: Mental clarity and emotional balance

Type: Layering Method

Ingredients:
- 1 drop Copaiba
- 1 drop Valor®
- 1 drop Sacred Frankincense™
- 1 drop Vetiver
- 1 drop Peppermint
- Carrier oil

Directions: Rub the oils one at a time on the back of the neck in a clockwise rotation. If you have sensitive skin, start by rubbing 2 drops of carrier oil, such as V-6™ or Grapeseed. Start with the first oil by dripping it on the back of the neck and rubbing it for 30 seconds. Continue this method with each oil, in the above order, finishing off with a little carrier oil.

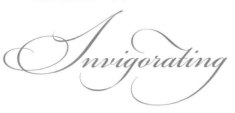

Invigorating

Supports: Heightened awareness

Type: Cold-water Diffuser Blend

Ingredients:

Recipe #1:
- 3 drops Ginger
- 3 drops Lemongrass

Recipe #2:
- 4 drops Into the Future™
- 3 drops Peppermint

Directions:
Add oils to cold-water diffuser and diffuse for 2-4 hours.

NOTE: You may convert this recipe to a 5mL rollerball. Triple the recipe and combine all essential oils into a 5mL rollerball bottle, swirl to blend, and let synergize for 24 hours before topping off with V-6™ or Fractionated Coconut carrier oil. Apply on wrists and back of neck as needed.

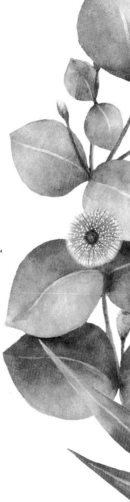

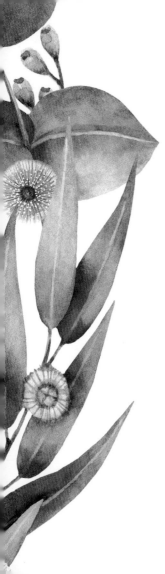

SPOTLIGHT ON RAVINTSARA

The single species oil called Ravintsara is commonly mistaken for Ravensara. Ravintsara is "ho leaf" oil from Madagascar. It's a little confusing because its official name with the Latin binomial is Chinese *Cinnamomum camphora* leaf oil, and it is also called "camphor." It's the oil in the newly reformulated Valor®. The identity thief known as Ravensara (*Ravensara aromatic*) is shrouded in a cloud of confusion as to where the name came from and what it actually is, but what we do know is it is also from the Lauraceae family from Madagascar, which is reported to contain over 30 species. Fantastic! That doesn't help narrow it down. We do know that it is different and has a mild camphor aroma compared to Ravintsara, which has a more pungent camphor aroma. Most consider it similar to Ravintsara, but you'll most likely never see actual Ravensara sold by anyone, even if it is labeled as such. If you have a bottle, it is most likely mislabeled and has Ravintsara inside. You'll most often see Ravensara cross-referenced with, or even placed in, the description of Ravintsara. Many authors mistakenly have the primary aromatic components for Ravintsara listed incorrectly under Ravensara. It is noted by listing Ravensara as having high percentages of Oxides (1,8 cineole), which is actually only found in Ravintsara. To make it more confusing, Young Living has a blend called Raven™ that contains mostly Ravintsara, along with Lemon, Wintergreen, Peppermint, and Eucalyptus radiata. Name confusion aside, this synergy is absolute magic! If you find yourself still confused, not to worry. The Ravintsara you have is a beautiful essential oil that is useful for calming and creating an open feeling when you breathe. Enjoy it, friend, and use it well! Below are the primary aromatic components of each oil.

RAVINTSARA
- 1,8 cineole (55+%)
- Monoterpenes (30%) in the form of:
  - sabinene (9-16%)
  - α-terpinene (5-10%)
  - α-pinene (4-6%)
- Plus others below 5%

RAVENSARA
- limonene (19%)
- sabinene (11%)
- methyl chavicol (8%)
- α-pinene (6%)
- plus others below 5%

SECTION THREE

PHYSICAL HEALTH

Recipes

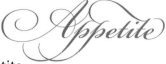

Supports: Healthy appetite

Type: Topical Rollerball

Ingredients:

Recipe #1:
- 20 drops Peppermint
- 10 drops Bergamot
- 5 drops Nutmeg
- Carrier oil

Recipe #2:
- 15 drops Ginger
- 10 drops Peppermint
- 3 drops Hyssop
- Carrier oil

Recipe #3:
- 10 drops Peppermint
- 10 drops Orange
- 5 drops Spearmint
- Carrier oil

Recipe #4:
- 10 drops Lemon
- 8 drops Black Pepper
- 5 drops Peppermint
- Carrier oil

Directions: Combine all essential oils to create a synergy in a 5mL rollerball and swirl bottle to mix well. It is suggested to let sit for 24 hours to fully synergize and then top off with V-6™ carrier oil or carrier of your choosing. Apply to your wrists and smell frequently during the day. Apply directly under your earlobe where it meets your jawline and in the crease on the back of your knees.

Armpit Serums

Type: Topical Rollerball or Dropper Serum

Ingredients:

Recipe #1
- 60 drops Purification®
- 20 drops Cypress
- 50 drops Jojoba oil

Recipe #2:
- 60 drops Tea Tree
- 30 drops Lavender
- 20 drops Cypress
- 50 drops Jojoba oil

Recipe #3:
- 40 drops Tea Tree
- 20 drops Geranium
- 20 drops Cypress
- 10 drops Lavender
- 50 drops Jojoba oil

Directions: Create a synergy of your desired essential oil recipe in a 15mL rollerball or dropper bottle and swirl bottle to mix well. Add 50 drops Jojoba oil. Jojoba is the only carrier that will not stain your clothing. Apply to clean armpits in the morning. Add more or less carrier oil to your liking.

Breast Health

Supports: Healthy breasts

Type: Rollerball

Ingredients:
Recipe #1:
- 10 drops Frankincense
- 5 drops Rosemary
- 5 drops Lavender
- Carrier oil

Recipe #2:
- 10 drops Clary Sage
- 8 drops Cypress
- 3 drops Geranium
- Carrier oil

Directions: Combine ingredients into a 5mL rollerball, swirl to blend, and let fully synergize for 24 hours, then top off with V-6™ carrier oil. Rub on breasts daily.

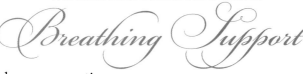

Breathing Support

Supports: Easy breezy sensation

Type: Topical Rollerball or Dropper (These are low dilution ratio recipes - cut recipes in half for those who are younger or more sensitive.)

Ingredients:

Recipe #1:
- 20 drops Lavender
- 20 drops Lemon
- 20 drops Peppermint
- Carrier oil

Recipe #2:
- 10 drops Raven™
- 5 drops Clove
- 5 drops Melaleuca Quinquenervia
- Carrier oil

Recipe #3:
- 40 drops Frankincense
- 20 drops Ravintsara
- 15 drops Clove
- 10 drops Myrrh
- 5 drops Sage
- Carrier oil

Directions: Add essential oils to a 15mL dropper or rollerball bottle, swirl to blend, and let synergize for 24 hours, then top off with carrier oil. Recipe #1: Rub 3–4 drops of the blend on your skull behind your ears and along your jawline on both sides of your head. Do this 2–4 times per day as needed. Recipes #2 & 3: Rub onto chest and back 3-4 times per day. Gently cup the area with your hand by patting the area with a cupped hand.

Bugs - Summertime

Supports: Outdoor nuisances

Type: Topical Dropper

Ingredients:
- 40 drops Tea Tree
- 20 drops Citronella
- 20 drops Lemongrass
- 20 drops Clove
- 20 drops Melaleuca Quinquenervia
- Carrier oil

Directions: Combine ingredients into a 15mL rollerball, swirl to blend, or let fully synergize for 24 hours, then top off with V-6™ carrier oil. Rub all over exposed skin every 4 hours.

Bugs - Outdoors

Supports: Outdoor nuisances

Type: Single Drop Application

Ingredients: (choose one of the following)
- 1 drop Purification®
- 1 drop Melrose™
- 1 drop Australian Kuranya™

Directions: Place one drop of undiluted essential oil on the bottom of your feet and rub in well every day. Apply this 20 minutes before going outside. If going to an area with a larger population of critters, apply a 50-50 mix of essential oil and carrier oil onto exposed skin. If hiking or doing stimulating activity, reapply every 2 hours. For normal support at work or school, this method will last 4-6 hours. Note: Do not use Purification® where bees are present. Bees are attracted to Lemongrass, one of the ingredients of Purification®.

Eye Area Serums

Supports: Smooth skin around the eye area

Type: Serum

Ingredients:

Recipe #1: (Basic Smoothing)
- 10 drops Frankincense
- 10 drops Myrrh

Recipe #2: (No Crow Smoothing)
- 15 drops Gentle Baby™
- 10 drops Sacred Frankincense™
- 10 drops Myrrh
- 6 drops Patchouli
- 2 drops Rose (optional)
- 2 drops Hyssop (optional)

Recipe #3: (Sight Support)
- 10 drops Frankincense
- 5 drops Copaiba
- 5 drops Lavender
- 5 drops Lemongrass
- 4 drops Helichrysum
- 2 drops Juniper

Recipe #4: (Health)
- 10 drops Tea Tree
- 10 drops Eucalyptus Radiata
- 10 drops Cypress

Directions: Combine all essential oils into a 5mL dropper bottle, swirl to blend, and let synergize for 24 hours. Top off with equal parts Jojoba and Jamaican Black Castor oils. Drip 2-5 drops into your palm, dip your ring finger into the serum, and dab all around eye area at night about 1 hour before bed. Pat off excess with a warm washcloth just before bed to avoid staining pillow case.

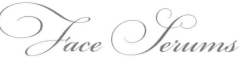

Face Serums

Supports: Smooth facial skin

Type: Serum

Ingredients:

Recipe #1 (Deluxe)
- 10 drops Frankincense
- 10 drops Lavender
- 10 drops Copaiba

Recipe #2: (Blemish)
- 10 drops Frankincense
- 10 drops Lavender
- 5 drops Tea Tree
- 5 drops Cedarwood

Recipe #3 (Sacred Seven)
- 7 drops Sacred Frankincense™
- 7 drops Frankincense
- 7 drops Sacred Sandalwood™
- 7 drops Myrrh
- 7 drops Cedarwood
- 7 drops Hyssop
- 7 drops Onycha

Recipe #4: (Pore Diminishing)
- 10 drops Frankincense
- 10 drops Lavender
- 10 drops Patchouli
- 10 drops Cedarwood
- 5 drops Jasmine

Directions: Combine all essential oils into a 15mL orifice reducer bottle, swirl to blend, and let synergize for 24 hours. Top off with carrier oil of your choice such as Rosehip Seed, which is one of the best for your face. Drip 2-5 drops into your palm, rub hands together, then apply all over your face, neck, chest, and back of hands morning and night. These serums may be used instead of your face creams.

Hair Serums

Supports: Shiny silky hair

Type: Neat Serum

Ingredients:

Recipe #1:
- 10 drops Frankincense
- 10 drops Rosemary
- 5 drops Lavender
- 5 drops Cedarwood
- 5 drops Sage

Recipe #2:
- 15 drops Frankincense
- 8 drops Lavender
- 8 drops Copaiba

Recipe #3:
- 10 drops Clary Sage
- 5 drops Copaiba
- 5 drops Frankincense
- 5 drops Rosemary
- 5 drops Lavender
- 5 drops Cedarwood

Recipe #4:
- 10 drops Lavender
- 10 drops Cedarwood

Directions: Combine all essential oils into a 5mL orifice reducer bottle, swirl to blend, and let synergize for 24 hours. Drip 2-5 drops into your palm, rub hands together, then apply to damp hair after you shower focusing on the middle of the shaft to the tips. Apply a pea size amount of leave-in conditioner to hair such as Copaiba Vanilla Moisturizing Conditioner™ from Young Living®.

Head Health

Supports: General health of the head

Type: Topical Layering

Ingredients:
- 1 drop Sacred Frankincense™
- 1 drop Helichrysum
- 1 drop Ledum
- 1 drop Sacred Sandalwood™
- 1 drop Melissa
- Carrier oil

Directions: Rub the oils one at a time over your heart in a clockwise rotation. If you have sensitive skin, start by rubbing 3 drops of carrier oil, such as V-6™ or Grapeseed. Start with the first oil by dripping it on your hand and then rubbing it on the back of the neck for 30 seconds. Continue this method with each oil in the above order. Finally, hold your hand on the back of your neck for an additional minute, casing in the oils.

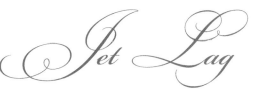

Jet Lag

Supports: Changing time zones with minimal issues

- SUPER HYDRATE: Up your water game at least one week prior to departure. Drink 80-100 ounces per day for 7 days prior to your trip. Continue to super hydrate during your trip as well. One drop of Tangerine Vitality™ and one drop of Peppermint Vitality™ in a 20 ounce glass or stainless steel water bottle is helpful during flights for nausea.

- NO SUGAR: Stop all processed sugar consumption (table sugar and added sugar items) for one week prior to trip. Fresh fruit is fine and encouraged.

- TIME RESET: When you get to the departure gate, set your watch to the arriving city's time. Note the hour and get your mind onto that time right away. If your flight is long, sleep on the plane when you would normally go to bed and stay awake at all costs during times that you should be awake. Do not nap!

- SLEEP: Use ImmuPro™ or SleepEssence™ to get your body to sleep. Apply a drop of Lavender with carrier into belly button.

- ANTI-OXIDATE: Drink 2-4 NingXia Red® packets per day during transition days and 1-2 during the regular days at your destination and again when you return home.

- NO NAPPING: Drink 1-2 NingXia Nitro® tubes to stay awake when you are tempted to nap during the day. Remember, do not nap.

- MOVE: During long flights, when you are supposed to be awake, move around the plane to get your lymphatic system moving. Do laps. When you get to the lavatory area, stretch your arms and legs with simple stretching techniques. Take 10 minutes every hour to do this. Do not worry about disturbing your seat mates. It's best to request an aisle seat during long flights for this reason.

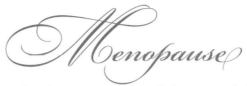

Menopause

Supports: Various needs when going through hormonal change

Ingredients:
Part 1: Hormone Support
- 1 drop Progessence Plus™

Part 2: Hormone and Hot Flash Support
- 10 drops Peppermint
- 3 drops Lime
- 3 drops Lavender
- 3 drops Clary Sage
- Water for Spritzer or Carrier oil for Roll-on

Part 3: Sleep Support
- 1-2 tablets ImmuPro™
Diffuser Blend:
- 3 drops Frankincense
- 3 drops Lavender
- 3 drops Cedarwood
Topical: (choose one)
- 1 drop Peace & Calming® on big toes
- 1 drop Valerian on big toes

Directions:

Part 1: Apply one drop of Progessence Plus™ morning and night on inner crease of elbows and front and back of neck.

Part 2: Combine all essential oils in a 4 ounce glass spray bottle and swirl to blend. Top off with alkaline water. Mist body as needed, keeping clear of face and eyes. Note: you may create a Roll-on by using a 5mL bottle. Add all essential oils to the bottle, swirl to blend, wait 24 hours to fully synergize, and then top off with V-6™ or Fractionated Coconut Carrier oil. Use a metal Rollerball fitment. Rub on back of neck, shoulders, chest, and on both feet below the inner and outer ankle bone as needed.

Part 3: As you get into bed: Apply the drop of Progessence Plus™ as noted above. Take 1-2 tablets of ImmuPro™. Set diffuser and run for 4 hours during sleep time. Apply one drop of Peace & Calming® or Valerian to your big toes. Have Spritzer bottle at bedside table in case of night sweats.

Motion Balance

Supports: For balancing when you are on a plane or boat

Type: Topical Roll-on

Ingredients:
- 10 drops Northern Lights Black Spruce™
- 8 drops Tangerine
- 5 drops Frankincense
- 5 drops Peppermint
- 2 drops Ginger
- Carrier oil

Directions: Add all essential oils to a 5mL bottle with a metal roller fitment. Swirl to blend, and allow to synergize for 24 hours. Top off with Carrier oil of your choice. Rub onto wrists first. Next, rub some on the tips of your fingers and apply all over ears, front and back, including the frontal lobe called the tragus. Do not get any into your inner ear.

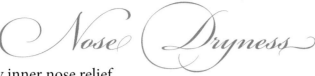

Nose Dryness

Supports: Dry inner nose relief

Type: Serum

Ingredients:

Recipe #1:
- 10 drops Myrrh
- 8 drops Elemi
- 5 drops Patchouli
- 5 drops Lavender
- 3 drops Neroli (optional)
- Jojoba Carrier oil

Recipe #2:
- 10 drops Lavender
- 10 drops Frankincense
- Jojoba Carrier oil

Recipe #3:
- 8 drops Frankincense
- 8 drops Lavender
- 8 drops Cedarwood
- 3 drops Geranium
- 2 drops Helichrysum
- Jojoba Carrier oil

Recipe #4:
- 10 drops Myrrh
- 8 drops Copaiba
- 5 drops Eucalyptus Radiata
- Jojoba Carrier oil

Directions: Add all essential oils to a 15mL glass dropper bottle. Swirl to blend, and let synergize for 24 hours. Fill dropper bottle half way with Jojoba carrier oil. Swirl to blend. Coat pinky finger with serum and rub inside the nostrils morning and evening.

Nail Beds

Supports: Healthy nail beds

Type: Layering

Ingredients:

Recipe #1:
- Lemon
- Frankincense
- Lavender
- Carrier oil

Recipe #2:
- Copaiba
- Kunzea
- Lemon
- Rosemary
- Carrier oil

Directions: Every night before bed, blend 2 drops of carrier oil and 1 drop of Lemon essential oil in the palm of your hand and rub onto each nail bed for 15 seconds each. Follow by using the same method with each oil in the above order. Each time, add 2 drops of carrier oil and 1 drop of essential oil, swirl in a clockwise motion with your massaging finger, then apply to each nail and massage it in fully.

Oola Balance™

Supports: "Designed to align and balance your center for a positive outlook and amplify the ability to focus on passions, behaviors, and health when diffused."
- Young Living®

Topical Support: Mental and emotional balance

Type: Diffuse or use as a Single Drop Application

Ingredient:
- Oola Balance™

Directions: Diffuse or apply Oola Balance™ on your wrists or drip one drop on the crown of your head to give you a feeling of focus and mental stability.

Tip: When applying this oil, state out loud the following: "I am fully aware of and at peace with my surroundings."

THE RECIPE BOOK *with Jen O'Sullivan*

Oola Family™

Supports: "Feelings of unconditional love, patience, and respect."

Topical Support: For emotional energy balance between you and other people

> Type: Diffuse or use as a Single Drop Application
>
> Ingredient:
> • Oola Family™

Directions: Diffuse or apply Oola Family™ on the back of your neck and one drop in your belly button in the morning to help with vibrational connections. This will help balance your emotions around others.

Tip: When applying this oil, state out loud the following: "I am unconditionally loving, patient, and respectful."

*Quoted text is from YoungLiving.com

74

Oola Faith™

Supports: "Enhances spiritual influences, promoting deeper meditation and a greater sense of spiritual awareness and connectedness."

Topical Support: For grounding and feelings of emotional security

Type: Diffuse or use as a Single Drop Application

Ingredient:
- Oola Faith™

Directions: Diffuse or apply Oola Faith™ on your wrists or drip one drop on the crown of your head to give you a feeling of being grounded and secure when going into public or to a party where you may be nervous.

Tip: When applying this oil, state out loud the following: "I am grateful, humble, and fully connected."

*Quoted text is from YoungLiving.com

Oola Field™

Supports: "Feelings of self-worth and strength that may help you reach your true, unlimited potential."

Topical Support: For clarity of mind and stimulation of muscles.

Type: Diffuse or use as a Single Drop Application

Ingredient:
- Oola Field™

Directions: Diffuse or apply Oola Field™ on the back of the neck for greater clarity and stimulation. Use this oil as a general pick-me-up during the day. Rub onto muscles before or after a strenuous workout.

Tip: When applying this oil, state out loud the following:
"I am pursuing my purpose in life."

*Quoted text is from YoungLiving.com

Oola Finance™

Supports: "Positive emotions and increased feelings of abundance."

Topical Support: For grounding and courage with a sense of resolve to move forward

Type: Diffuse or use as a Single Drop Application

Ingredient:
• Oola Finance™

Directions: Diffuse or apply Oola Finance™ on your wrists and front of neck or apply one drop to the top of your head on your scalp and some to the arches of your feet in the morning before you start your day. This will help you feel grounded and motivated.

Tip: When applying this oil, state out loud the following: "I am financially free and living abundantly."

*Quoted text is from YoungLiving.com

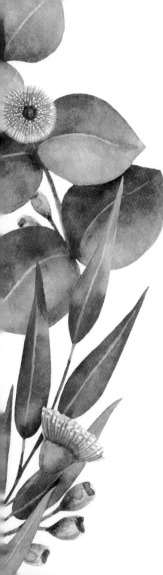

Oola Fitness™

Supports: "Specially formulated to uplift, energize, and give you the inspiration to set and achieve your strength and fitness goals."

Topical Support: For muscle support before and after a workout

Type: Diffuse or use as a Single Drop Application

Ingredient:
- Oola Fitness™

Directions: Diffuse or apply Oola Fitness™ directly on areas that need support before a strenuous workout. Following your workout, apply again to the same area.

Tip: When applying this oil, state out loud the following: "I am fit, healthy, disciplined, and strong."

*Quoted text is from YoungLiving.com

Oola Friends™

Supports: "Feelings of self-worth, empowerment, confidence, and awareness."

Topical Support: For focus while studying or needing extra concentration

Type: Diffuse or use as a Single Drop Application

Ingredient:
- Oola Friends™

Directions: Diffuse or apply Oola Friends™ to the back of your neck and wrists during a study session or time of needed clarity and focus.

Tip: When applying this oil, state out loud the following:
"I am blessed with empowering, healthy relationships."

*Quoted text is from YoungLiving.com

Oola Fun™

Supports: "Boosts self-confidence to impart a positive outlook that can enhance the pleasure of pursuing the joys of life."

Topical Support: For thigh skin tightening and smoothing

Type: Diffuse or use as a Multiple Drop Application

Ingredient:
- Oola Fun™

Directions: Diffuse as is, or apply Oola Fun™ directly and liberally using a carrier oil on your thighs morning and night. Avoid using in the morning if sunbathing that day.

Tip: When applying this oil, state out loud the following:
"I am pursuing the joys of life."

*Quoted text is from YoungLiving.com

Oola Grow™

Supports: "Gives you courage to focus on the task at hand and helps you move toward positive advancement and progression." - Young Living®

Topical Support: Bedroom intimacy

Type: Diffuse or use as a Single Drop Application

Ingredient:
• Oola Grow™

Directions: Diffuse or apply Oola Grow™ to your inner thighs just before intimacy to increase sensuality and to help support an emotional connection with your partner.

Tip: When applying this oil, state out loud the following: "I am strong, confident, and successful."

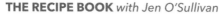

Respiration

Supports: For open airway feeling

Type: Steam Bowl

Ingredients:
Recipe #1:
- 3 drops Raven™
- 1 drop Peppermint
- 1 drop Lavender

Recipe #1:
- 3 drops RC™
- 1 drop Cypress
- 1 drop Pine

Directions: Fill a large mixing bowl with boiling water. Add essential oils to the water, close eyes, and place head over the steam. Breathe in deeply for 3-5 minutes. If desired, place a towel or cloth over your head to case in the steam.

Scalp Itch

Supports: For occasional scalp itch relief

Type: Spritzer

Ingredients:

Recipe #1:
- 10 drops Manuka
- 10 drops Peppermint
- 5 drops Frankincense
- 5 drops Tea Tree
- 5 drops Rosemary
- Distilled water

Recipe #2:
- 10 drops Peppermint
- 10 drops Cypress
- 10 drops Tea Tree
- 5 drops Rosemary
- 5 drops Lavender
- Distilled water

Directions: Add all essential oils to a 4 ounce glass spray bottle. Swirl to blend, and let synergize for 24 hours. Top off with distilled water, shake well, and spray liberally onto towel-dried scalp after your shower.

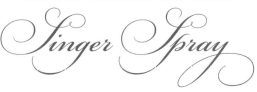

Supports: Calming of the neck and larynx

Type: Throat Spray

Ingredients:

Recipe #1:
- 10 drops Frankincense
- 10 drops Copaiba
- 5 drops Eucalyptus Radiata
- 2 drops Thyme

Recipe #2:
- 10 drops Frankincense
- 5 drops Lavender
- 5 drops Bergamot

Directions: Add essential oils to a 2 ounce glass spray bottle. Swirl to blend, and let synergize for 24 hours. Add a pinch of Pink Himalayan Sea Salt. Fill with distilled water. Spray on back of throat and front of neck as needed.

Type: Single Drop Method

Ingredients: (choose one of the following)
- 1 drop Frankincense
- 1 drop Sacred Sandalwood™

Directions: Apply directly to the front of the neck just before singing.

Skin Support

Supports: Skin smoothing

Type: Serum

Ingredients:

Recipe #1:
- 10 drops Frankincense
- 10 drops Lavender
- 10 drops Copaiba

Recipe #2:
- 10 drops Frankincense
- 8 drops Lavender
- 5 drops Manuka
- 3 drops Blue Tansy
- 2 drops Carrot Seed

Recipe #3:
- 10 drops Sacred Sandalwood™
- 8 drops Patchouli
- 5 drops Cedarwood

Recipe #4:
- 10 drops Myrrh
- 10 drops Frankincense
- 4 drops Gentle Baby™
- 5 drops Hyssop

Directions: Create a synergy of your desired essential oil recipe in a 15mL dropper bottle. Swirl to blend, and let synergize for 24 hours. Top off with carrier oil and apply to face, neck, chest, and back of hands morning and night. Use this instead of traditional face creams. Carrier oils to consider: Grapeseed, Rosehip Seed, Sweet Almond, Mustard Seed, or your favorite skin nourishing carrier oil.

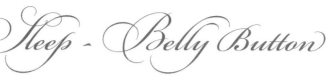

Sleep - Belly Button

Supports: More restful sleep

Type: Single Belly Button Drop Application

Ingredients: (choose one of the following:)
- Lavender
- Stress Away™
- Valor®
- Peace & Calming®
- Sandalwood
- Frankincense
- Copaiba

Directions: Lie down on your back and drip one drop of carrier oil directly into your belly button followed by one of the above essential oils. Drip a drop or two of carrier oil such as V-6™, Grapeseed, or Mustard seed directly on top of the essential oil. Lie still on your back for at least 20 minutes. Use a cotton ball to keep oil from leaking out onto your sheets.

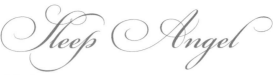

Supports: More restful sleep

Type: Topical Rollerball or diffuser blend

Ingredients:

Recipe #1:
- 8 drops Valor®
- 6 drops Roman Chamomile

Recipe #2:
- 6 drops Patchouli
- 6 drops Tangerine

Recipe #3:
- 3 drops Stress Away™
- 3 drops Sacred Sandalwood™

Recipe #4:
- 6 drops Peace & Calming®
- 4 drops Frankincense
- 2 drops Vetiver

Recipe #5:
- 6 drops Sacred Sandalwood™
- 3 drops Lime

Recipe #6:
- 6 drops Bergamot
- 6 drops Cedarwood

Directions: Combine all essential oils into a 5mL rollerball bottle, swirl to blend, and let synergize for 24 hours before topping off with V-6™ or Fractionated Coconut carrier oil. Apply on wrists, back of neck, and across forehead just before going to bed. Note: Convert this recipe to a diffuser blend by adding half the above drops into a cold-water diffuser.

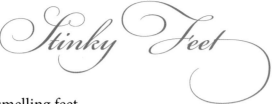

Stinky Feet

Supports: Fresh-smelling feet

Type: Single Drop Application

Ingredients: (choose one of the following)
- Purification®
- Melrose™
- Australian Kuranya™
- Tea Tree

Directions: Drip one drop of one of the above oils directly onto the bottom of your freshly cleansed foot and rub together with the other foot. Another option is to use your hand and rub the oil directly onto the bottom of your feet, covering the entire pad and in between toes. Do this just before you put on your shoes.

Tender Tendons

Supports: Healthy tendons and ligaments

Type: Layering Method

Ingredients:
- 1 drop Copaiba
- 1 drop PanAway®
- 3 drops Lemongrass
- Carrier oil

Directions: Rub the oils, one at a time, directly on the desired area. If you have sensitive skin, start by rubbing 2 drops of carrier oil, such as V-6™ or Grapeseed onto the area. Start with the first oil and drip it into your hand, then rub it in small clockwise circular motions on the location. Continue this method with each oil in the above order and finishing off with a little carrier oil.

Withdrawal Protocol

30 Day Withdrawal Protocol: To be followed for a minimum of 30 days.

This is not a diet. It is meant to support your body when you remove something from your life that you are physically addicted to such as coffee, nicotine, grains, dairy, drugs, etc. Eat normally but try to get more fruits and veggies and less processed foods.

Stop all caffeine consumption. No coffee, no decaf, no tea (herbal is fine), no caffeinated sodas, no chocolate, no Excedrin® or pills containing caffeine. For a warm cup morning routine, try Dandy Blend Instant Herbal Beverage with Dandelion. It's a great healthy substitute!

Drink 2 ounces of NingXia Red® 4 times per day for the first week and then adjust down to 2 times per day or as needed.

Drink lots of alkaline water; at least half your body weight in ounces. Example: if you weigh 200 lbs then divide 200 by 2 to get 100, change lbs to ounces, and this will give you your daily intake being 100 ounces. Use 1-3 drops per day of your favorite Vitality™ citrus essential oil single or blend.

Juice at least once per day, and twice if you can. Masticating juicers are best, but a centrifugal juicer is fine too. Drink 12-16 ounces of juiced dark leafy greens such as kale and spinach. Add cucumber, celery, and green apples. Use fresh ginger too if you are experiencing nausea. Drink within 15 minutes of creation to obtain the most benefits.

Take a hot bath every night with 2 cups Epsom Salt and 2 cups Dead Sea Salt for the first 7 nights. For the remainder of the detox, take 2-4 baths per week.

The first week get a Raindrop Technique® massage. Drink more water than usual on this day after your session. Then get a circulation enhancing deep tissue massage once a week. These are often called sports massage to encourage blood flow.

Exercise for a minimum of 30 minutes per day. A brisk walk is fine. You must maintain a higher heart rate and should be sweating by 10 minutes into the exercise. If you're able to freely talk to someone then you're not trying hard enough. You must get your lymphatic system moving.

Give yourself freedom to nap and sleep longer. If sleeping in is not an option, then make sure you go to sleep 2 hours earlier than normal.

Expect to be crabby! Your body won't be happy but it's important to stick with this for the full 30 days. Mood swings and a gory temper are to be expected. Use your favorite emotion supporting oils such as Valor®, Melissa, Stress Away™, or Sandalwood.

Products to use on this protocol: NingXia Red® to cleanse, AlkaLime® for pH balance, Vitality™ Citrus oils to cleanse, ImmuPro™ or SleepEssence™ for sleep training, MightyPro™ and/or Life 9™ for gut health, Super B™ for energy, and Super Cal Plus™ for calcium and vital Vitamin D3.

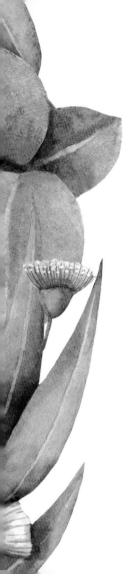

SPOTLIGHT ON MELALEUCA

Tea Tree (*Melaleuca alternifolia*) and Niaouli (*Melaleuca quinquernervia*)often get called the two different versions of Tea Trees. Technically, only Melaleuca alternifolia has the common name Tea Tree, while Melaleuca quinquenervia is called Niaouli. They are both Melaleuca oils from the Myrtle family of trees. The term "alternifolia" means "having leaves that alternate on each side of a stem." The species is commonly called Narrow-leaf paperbark or Narrow-leaf Tea Tree. The genus is Melaleuca and the species is alternifolia. Tea Tree is high in the monoterpene terpinen-4-ol (also high in Nutmeg). In the case of Melaleuca quinquenervia, the family is also from the Myrtle (Myrtaceae), and the genus is Melaleuca, but the species is quinquenervia. The tree is commonly called Broad-leaved Paperbark or Broad-leaved Tea Tree. The term "quinquenervia" is from the Latin meaning "five nerves" as the leaves of the tree have 5 veins. Its common name in the United States is Punk Tree. I think the oil should be called Punk, don't you? The actual common name is Niaouli. Niaouli is high in the Monoterpene Oxide 1,8 Cineole, which is commonly known as Eucalyptol (found in Eucalyptus). The similarities to these oils stop at their names. When you take a closer look at their molecular profiles, you will learn quickly how very different they are. Homework: Go to Wikipedia and look up two things: terpinen-4-ol and 1,8 cineole. This will give you the clear answer on how these oils are different. Let's take a look:

MELALEUCA ALTERNIFOLIA
High in Monoterpenes (70-90%)
- terpinen-4-ol (40%)
- γ-terpinene (20%)
- α-terpinene (10%)
- 1,8 cineole (5-15%)
- α-pinene (5%)

MELALEUCA QUINQUENERVIA
High in Monoterpene Oxides (60+%)
- 1,8 cineole (55-75%)
- α-pinene (5-12%)
- Viridiflorol (2-6%)
- Limonene (1-9%)

CHILDREN & DOGS

Recipes

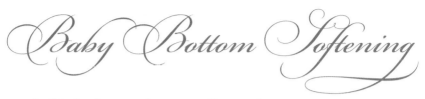

Baby Bottom Softening

Supports: Soft baby bottom between diaper changes

Type: Topical Dropper Serum

Ingredients:

Recipe #1:
- 20 drops Gentle Baby™
- 10 drops Elemi
- 5 drops Patchouli
- Carrier oil

Recipe #2:
- 20 drops Geranium
- 20 drops Lavender
- 20 drops Cedarwood
- 15 drops Roman Chamomile
- 5 drops Jasmine
- Carrier oil

Directions: Add essential oils to a 15mL dropper bottle, swirl to blend, let synergize for 24 hours, and then top off with V-6™ carrier oil, Fractionated Coconut oil, or Grapeseed oil. Apply during diaper changes.

Bed Wetting

Supports: Bladder control through the night

Type: Topical Rollerball

Ingredients:
- 10 drops Cypress
- 5 drops Northern Lights Black Spruce™
- 5 drops Lavender
- Carrier oil

Directions: Add essential oils to a 5mL roller bottle, swirl to blend, let synergize for 24 hours, and then top off with V-6™ carrier oil or Fractionated Coconut oil. Rub directly onto abdomen before bed. Use for a minimum of 5 nights to start seeing results.

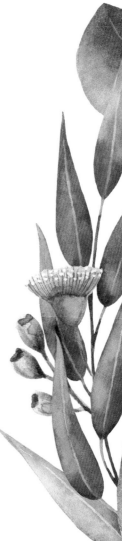

Bugs - School-Age Critters

Supports: Critter-free childhood

Type: Topical Single Drop Method

Ingredients: (use one of the following)
- 1 drop Purification®
- 1 drop Melrose™

Directions: Place one drop of undiluted Purification® on the bottom of your feet and rub in well every day. Apply this 20 minutes before going outside. If going to an area with a larger population of critters, apply a 50-50 mix of Purification® and carrier oil onto exposed skin. If hiking or doing stimulating activity, reapply every 2 hours. For normal support at work or school, this method will last 4-6 hours. For hair critters, rub a small amount of Purification® onto your hands and then apply to the back of the hairline without touching the skin.

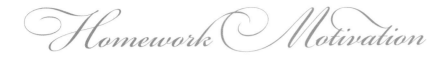

Homework Motivation

Supports: Encourages focus and motivation

Type: Topical Rollerball

Ingredients:

Recipe #1:

- 10 drops Peppermint
- 5 drops Motivation™
- 2 drops Vetiver

Recipe #2:

- 10 drops Magnify Your Purpose™
- 8 drops Wintergreen
- 5 drops Lemon

Directions: Add essential oils to a 5mL roller bottle, swirl to blend, let synergize for 24 hours, and then top off with V-6™ carrier oil or Fractionated Coconut oil. Rub onto wrists and back of neck. Create a diffuser blend by adding 4-6 drops of the synergy to your cold-water diffuser.

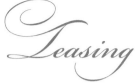

Teasing

Supports: Feelings of courage and calm

Type: Layering Method

Ingredients:
- 1 drop Northern Lights Black Spruce™
- 1 drop Copaiba
- 1 drop Frankincense
- 1 drop Pine
- 1 drop Vetiver
- 1 drop Peppermint

Directions: Start by dripping one drop of Northern Lights Black Spruce™ directly on the top of the scalp at the uppermost part while standing up by parting the hair to drip it directly on the skin. Next, rub the oils one at a time directly over the heart in a clockwise circular motion. If you have sensitive skin, start by rubbing 2 drops of carrier oil, such as V-6™ or Grapeseed. Continue this method with each oil in the above order, finishing off with a little carrier oil.

NOTE: You may convert this recipe to a 5mL rollerball. Double or triple the recipe to your liking and combine all essential oils into a 5mL rollerball bottle, swirl to blend, and let synergize for 24 hours before topping off with V-6™ or Fractionated Coconut carrier oil. Apply on wrists and back of neck.

Temperature Support

Supports: Body temperature regulation

Type: Belly Button Drop Method

Ingredients:
- 1 drop Carrier oil
- 1 drop Peppermint
- 1 drop Lime

Directions: While lying on back, apply each drop, one at a time, directly onto or in the belly button in the above order. Remain still for 20 minutes or apply a cotton ball over belly button with tape to hold in place.

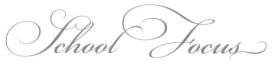

School Focus

Supports: Mental clarity and focus

Type: Single Drop Application

Ingredients: (use one of the following)
- Stress Away™
- Peace & Calming®
- Valor®
- GeneYus™
- Brain Power™
- Sacred Frankincense™
- Sacred Sandalwood™
- Northern Lights Black Spruce™

Directions: Apply a single drop on wrists and back of neck in the morning before school.

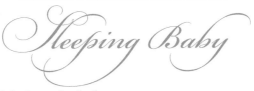

Supports: More restful sleep for baby

Type: Topical Rollerball or Diffuser Blend

Ingredients:

Recipe #1:
- 4 drops Gentle Baby™
- 4 drops Royal Hawaiian Sandalwood™

Recipe #2:
- 3 drops Valor®
- 2 drops Copaiba

Recipe #3:
- 4 drops Peace & Calming®
- 2 drops Tangerine

Recipe #4:
- 2 drops Frankincense
- 2 drops Vetiver
- 2 drops Lavender
- 2 drops Cedarwood

Recipe #5:
- 2 drops Gentle Baby™
- 2 drops Tangerine
- 2 drops Lemon Myrtle

Directions: Combine all essential oils into a 5mL rollerball bottle, swirl to blend, let synergize for 24 hours, and then top off with V-6™ or Fractionated Coconut carrier oil. Apply on bottom of feet and big toes before bedtime. Note: Convert this recipe to a diffuser blend by adding half the above drops into a cold-water diffuser.

Dog - Furniture Care

Supports: Keeping dogs off furniture and carpet

Type: Spray

Ingredients:
- 10 drops Tea Tree
- Vinegar
- Water

Directions: Add essential oil to an 8 ounce spray bottle. Fill half way with vinegar and the rest with tap water. Shake before each use. Spray on furniture or carpet that you want dogs to stay away from. Test a small area for color fastness before spraying a larger area. Caution spraying lacquered wood as Tea Tree is high in Monoterpenes and will dissolve synthetic coatings, plastics, and paint over prolonged use.

Dog - Lawn Care

Supports: Keeping dogs off lawns

Type: Spray

Ingredients:
- 6 drops Purification®
- 20 drops Neem Carrier oil (optional)
- Water

Directions: Add carrier oil and essential oil to an 8 ounce spray bottle (does not need to be glass). Fill with warm tap water and shake before each use. Spray on lawn in the morning at least 30 minutes after sprinklers have turned off. Spray the entire lawn area where dogs tend to relieve themselves.

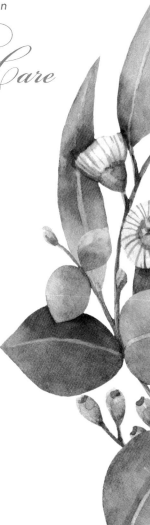

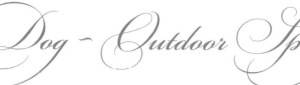

Dog - Outdoor Spray

Supports: A critter free fur-baby

Type: Spritzer

Ingredients:
Recipe #1:
- 3 drops Purification®
- 10 drops Neem Carrier oil

Recipe #2:
- 4 drops Cinnamon Bark
- 4 drops Cedarwood
- 4 drops Lavender
- 2 ounces Apple Cider Vinegar

Directions: Add carrier oil and essential oil to a 4 ounce glass spray bottle. Fill with tap water and shake before each use. Use before each outdoor walk. Spray lightly on paws, underbelly, and back, staying clear of the head area.

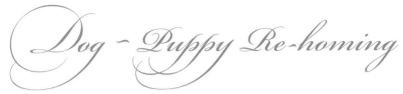

Dog ~ Puppy Re-homing

Supports: Bringing a new puppy home to help him or her adjust from not having mama around anymore

Type: Cold-water Diffuser Blend & Spritzer

Ingredients:
- 2 drops Copaiba
- 2 drops Frankincense
- 1 drop Lime
- 1 drop Cedarwood
- 1 drop Lavender

Directions: Use a cold-water diffuser. Add the essential oils one at a time directly on top of each other in the water or create a synergy by adding them to a clean dropper bottle, swirl to blend, allow to synergize for 24 hours, and then add 4 drops to your diffuser. Place diffuser in room with the puppy on the opposite side of the room. Play happily in a protected corner of the room. Have a soft blanket for the puppy to be on. Create a spritzer using the same above recipe in an 8 ounce glass spray bottle with water. At night, toss the puppy's blanket into the dryer for 10 minutes, pull it out, and spray the blanket on one side. Place it with the puppy to encourage sleep, warmth, and a healthy and happy smell memory.

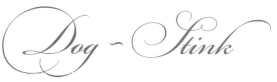

Supports: Fresh-smelling dog

Type: Spritzer

Ingredients:

Recipe #1:
- 5 drops Lavender
- 5 drops Cedarwood
- 3 drops Eucalyptus Radiata

Recipe #2:
- 5 drops Lavender
- 5 drops Cedarwood
- 2 ounces Apple Cider Vinegar

Recipe #3:
- 4 drops Northern Lights Black Spruce
- 3 drops Rosemary
- 3 drops Lavender

Recipe #4:
- 3 drops Lemongrass
- 3 drops Cinnamon Bark
- 3 drops Lavender

Directions: Add essential oils to a 4 ounce glass spray bottle and swirl to blend. Fill with tap water. Shake well before use. Mist lightly over dog's coat and underbelly, keeping clear of the head. Use Recipe #2 for a natural solution for outdoor critters.

Dog - Stress

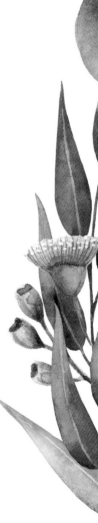

Supports: Feelings of calming and stabilizing

Type: Cold-water Diffuser Blend

Ingredients:

Recipe #1:
- 5 drops Peace & Calming®
- 2 drops Cedarwood

Recipe #2:
- 5 drops Copaiba
- 3 drops Cedarwood
- 2 drops Vetiver

Directions: Add oils to your cold-water diffuser and diffuse for 2-4 hours to help your dog stay calm. Allow ample open-air space for your pet to move to a different area.

NOTE: You may convert these recipes to a 5mL rollerball. Combine all essential oils into a 5mL rollerball bottle, swirl to blend, and let synergize for 24 hours before topping off with V-6™ or Fractionated Coconut carrier oil. Apply directly onto the pads of the feet, rub some on the back of the neck, or rub a little on the flaps of the ears.

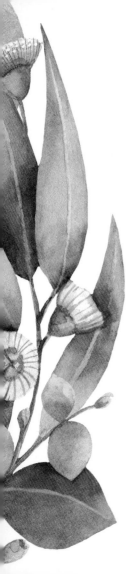

SPOTLIGHT ON JASMINE

Have you ever wondered why Jasmine may have a slight fecal aroma at times? Let's explore! Jasmine (*Jasminum*) comes from the Persian word "Yasameen," meaning "gift from God." There are over 100 different molecular constituents that make up Jasmine essential oil, with about 50% being in the Ester family. Esters are known for their calming, relaxing, and balancing properties. The primary esters found in Jasmine essential oil are benzyl acetate and benzyl benzoate, which are responsible for its fragrant floral aroma. Jasmine is known to support emotions, hormones, and your skin. It's amazing in face serums and is often used alone in a roller as a personal fragrance. It's strong, so you only need a small amount; 3-4 drops in a 5ml roller filled with carrier oil will be enough.

On the flip side of that glorious aroma that Jasmine is famous for is a dirty little molecule called "skatole." It's one of the constituents that is of smaller percentages in the oil, but it can be disconcerting when noticed. Have you noticed it? Scenario: You use Jasmine in the morning, and toward the end of the day you notice it, a faint, albeit distinct fecal smell. Yuck! Yep, it's your beloved Jasmine! What on Earth? Skatole is derived from the Greek root "skato-" which means "dung." You'll hear hunters refer to wild animal droppings as skat. Skatole in small amounts has a floral aroma, as in Jasmine. Once some of the lighter molecules wear off, the leftover skatole will only be noticed by the most discerning of noses, but it's definitely a fecal aroma.

Skatole is a base note that has a low volatility, which means it is the last molecule to leave the skin. Base notes help keep other molecules around longer, so you'll often see synthetic skatole used in perfumes. Don't let this deter you from purchasing this incredible little gem. One bottle will last you several years! Keep Jasmine out of direct sunlight. That includes your skin. The sun rays will cause the skatole to deteriorate faster and will give off its stronger dung aroma. When using this oil, apply it where the sun won't come in contact with it. For certain use it, though! It is amazing and very uncommon to notice the skatole.

SECTION FIVE

FRAGRANCE
Recipes

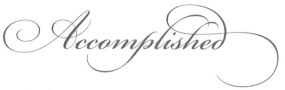

Supports: Home air freshener and personal fragrance for feelings of accomplishment

Type: Cold-water Diffuser Blend

Ingredients:
- 3 drops Lemon
- 2 drops Lemongrass
- 2 drops Tea Tree

Directions: Use a cold-water diffuser. Add the essential oils, one at a time directly on top of each other, in the water. You may also create a synergy. Add the oils to a clean dropper bottle, swirl to blend, and allow to synergize for 24 hours. Once synergized, add 4-12 drops to your diffuser.

NOTE: You may convert this recipe to a 5mL rollerball for a personal fragrance. Double or triple the recipe to your liking and combine all essential oils into a 5mL rollerball bottle, swirl to blend, and let synergize for 24 hours before topping off with V-6™ or Fractionated Coconut carrier oil. Apply on wrists and along sides of neck.

Awakened

Supports: Home air freshener and personal fragrance for feelings of emotional awakening

Type: Cold-water Diffuser Blend

Ingredients:
- 2 drops Awaken™
- 4 drops Grapefruit

Directions: Use a cold-water diffuser. Add the essential oils, one at a time directly on top of each other, in the water. You may also create a synergy. Add the oils to a clean dropper bottle, swirl to blend, and allow to synergize for 24 hours. Once synergized, add 4-12 drops to your diffuser.

NOTE: You may convert this recipe to a 5mL rollerball for a personal fragrance. Double or triple the recipe to your liking and combine all essential oils into a 5mL rollerball bottle, swirl to blend, and let synergize for 24 hours before topping off with V-6™ or Fractionated Coconut carrier oil. Apply on wrists and along sides of neck.

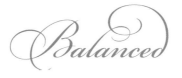

Balanced

Supports: Home air freshener and personal fragrance for feelings of emotional balance

Type: Cold-water Diffuser Blend

Ingredients:
- 3 drops Lavender
- 2 drops Clary Sage
- 2 drops Bergamot

Directions: Use a cold-water diffuser. Add the essential oils, one at a time directly on top of each other, in the water. You may also create a synergy. Add the oils to a clean dropper bottle, swirl to blend, and allow to synergize for 24 hours. Once synergized, add 4-12 drops to your diffuser.

NOTE: You may convert this recipe to a 5mL rollerball for a personal fragrance. Double or triple the recipe to your liking and combine all essential oils into a 5mL rollerball bottle, swirl to blend, and let synergize for 24 hours before topping off with V-6™ or Fractionated Coconut carrier oil. Apply on wrists and along sides of neck.

Burly Man

Supports: Home air freshener for men and personal fragrance for feelings of grounding and courage

Type: Cold-water Diffuser Blend

Ingredients:
- 5 drops Bergamot
- 3 drops Vetiver
- 3 drops Sacred Sandalwood™

Directions: Use a cold-water diffuser. Add the essential oils, one at a time directly on top of each other, in the water. You may also create a synergy. Add the oils to a clean dropper bottle, swirl to blend, and allow to synergize for 24 hours. Once synergized, add 4-12 drops to your diffuser.

NOTE: You may convert this recipe to a 5mL rollerball for a personal fragrance. Double or triple the recipe to your liking and combine all essential oils into a 5mL rollerball bottle, swirl to blend, and let synergize for 24 hours before topping off with V-6™ or Fractionated Coconut carrier oil. Apply on wrists and along sides of neck.

Calmed

Supports: Home air freshener and personal fragrance for feelings of emotional calming

Type: Cold-water Diffuser Blend

Ingredients:
- 2 drops Roman Chamomile
- 2 drops Lavender
- 2 drops Frankincense

Directions: Use a cold-water diffuser. Add the essential oils, one at a time directly on top of each other, in the water. You may also create a synergy. Add the oils to a clean dropper bottle, swirl to blend, and allow to synergize for 24 hours. Once synergized, add 4-12 drops to your diffuser.

NOTE: You may convert this recipe to a 5mL rollerball for a personal fragrance. Double or triple the recipe to your liking and combine all essential oils into a 5mL rollerball bottle, swirl to blend, and let synergize for 24 hours before topping off with V-6™ or Fractionated Coconut carrier oil. Apply on wrists and along sides of neck.

Chai Tea

Supports: Home air freshener and personal fragrance for feelings of security and family

Type: Cold-water Diffuser Blend

Ingredients:

- 3 drops Ginger
- 3 drops Orange
- 2 drops Cinnamon Bark
- 2 drops Clove

Directions: Use a cold-water diffuser. Add the essential oils, one at a time directly on top of each other, in the water. You may also create a synergy. Add the oils to a clean dropper bottle, swirl to blend, and allow to synergize for 24 hours. Once synergized, add 4-12 drops to your diffuser.

NOTE: You may convert this recipe to a 5mL rollerball for a personal fragrance. Double or triple the recipe to your liking and combine all essential oils into a 5mL rollerball bottle, swirl to blend, and let synergize for 24 hours before topping off with V-6™ or Fractionated Coconut carrier oil. Apply on wrists and along sides of neck.

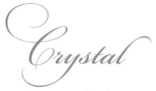

Crystal

Supports: Home air freshener and personal fragrance for feelings of emotional clarity of mind

Type: Cold-water Diffuser Blend

Ingredients:
- 6 drops Clarity™
- 2 drops Lemon

Directions: Use a cold-water diffuser. Add the essential oils, one at a time directly on top of each other, in the water. You may also create a synergy. Add the oils to a clean dropper bottle, swirl to blend, and allow to synergize for 24 hours. Once synergized, add 4-12 drops to your diffuser.

NOTE: You may convert this recipe to a 5mL rollerball for a personal fragrance. Double or triple the recipe to your liking and combine all essential oils into a 5mL rollerball bottle, swirl to blend, and let synergize for 24 hours before topping off with V-6™ or Fractionated Coconut carrier oil. Apply on wrists and along sides of neck.

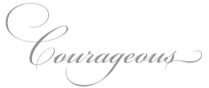

Courageous

Supports: Home air freshener and personal fragrance for feelings of emotional courage

Type: Cold-water Diffuser Blend

Ingredients:
- 4 drops Northern Lights Black Spruce™
- 2 drops Frankincense
- 2 drops Blue Tansy

Directions: Use a cold-water diffuser. Add the essential oils, one at a time directly on top of each other, in the water. You may also create a synergy. Add the oils to a clean dropper bottle, swirl to blend, and allow to synergize for 24 hours. Once synergized, add 4-12 drops to your diffuser.

NOTE: You may convert this recipe to a 5mL rollerball for a personal fragrance. Double or triple the recipe to your liking and combine all essential oils into a 5mL rollerball bottle, swirl to blend, and let synergize for 24 hours before topping off with V-6™ or Fractionated Coconut carrier oil. Apply on wrists and along sides of neck.

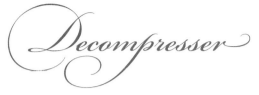

Decompresser

Supports: Home air freshener and personal fragrance for feelings of emotional decompression and stress relief

Type: Cold-water Diffuser Blend

Ingredients:
- 4 drops Copaiba
- 4 drops Lime
- 2 drops Lavender
- 2 drops Cedarwood
- 1 drop Patchouli

Directions: Use a cold-water diffuser. Add the essential oils, one at a time directly on top of each other, in the water. You may also create a synergy. Add the oils to a clean dropper bottle, swirl to blend, and allow to synergize for 24 hours. Once synergized, add 4-12 drops to your diffuser.

NOTE: You may convert this recipe to a 5mL rollerball for a personal fragrance. Double or triple the recipe to your liking and combine all essential oils into a 5mL rollerball bottle, swirl to blend, and let synergize for 24 hours before topping off with V-6™ or Fractionated Coconut carrier oil. Apply on wrists and along sides of neck.

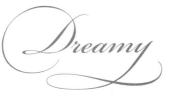

Supports: Home air freshener and personal fragrance for feelings of peace

Type: Cold-water Diffuser Blend

Ingredients:
- 3 drops Royal Hawaiian Sandalwood™
- 2 drops Tangerine

Directions: Use a cold-water diffuser. Add the essential oils, one at a time directly on top of each other, in the water. You may also create a synergy. Add the oils to a clean dropper bottle, swirl to blend, and allow to synergize for 24 hours. Once synergized, add 4-12 drops to your diffuser.

NOTE: You may convert this recipe to a 5mL rollerball for a personal fragrance. Double or triple the recipe to your liking and combine all essential oils into a 5mL rollerball bottle, swirl to blend, and let synergize for 24 hours before topping off with V-6™ or Fractionated Coconut carrier oil. Apply on wrists and along sides of neck.

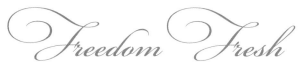

Freedom Fresh

Supports: Home air freshener and personal fragrance for feelings of youth and freedom

Type: Cold-water Diffuser Blend

Ingredients:
- 6 drops Grapefruit
- 2 drops Peppermint

Directions: Use a cold-water diffuser. Add the essential oils, one at a time directly on top of each other, in the water. You may also create a synergy. Add the oils to a clean dropper bottle, swirl to blend, and allow to synergize for 24 hours. Once synergized, add 4-12 drops to your diffuser.

NOTE: You may convert this recipe to a 5mL rollerball for a personal fragrance. Double or triple the recipe to your liking and combine all essential oils into a 5mL rollerball bottle, swirl to blend, and let synergize for 24 hours before topping off with V-6™ or Fractionated Coconut carrier oil. Apply on wrists and along sides of neck.

Fresh Air

Supports: Home air freshener and personal fragrance for feelings of openness when breathing

Type: Cold-water Diffuser Blend

Ingredients:
- 3 drops Peppermint
- 3 drops Lavender
- 3 drops Lemon

Directions: Use a cold-water diffuser. Add the essential oils, one at a time directly on top of each other, in the water. You may also create a synergy. Add the oils to a clean dropper bottle, swirl to blend, and allow to synergize for 24 hours. Once synergized, add 4-12 drops to your diffuser.

NOTE: You may convert this recipe to a 5mL rollerball for a personal fragrance. Double or triple the recipe to your liking and combine all essential oils into a 5mL rollerball bottle, swirl to blend, and let synergize for 24 hours before topping off with V-6™ or Fractionated Coconut carrier oil. Apply on wrists and along sides of neck and jawline.

Freshly Bright

Supports: Home air freshener and personal fragrance for feelings of calm and clear alertness

Type: Cold-water Diffuser Blend

Ingredients:
- 6 drops Lemon
- 4 drops Bergamot
- 4 drops Spearmint

Directions: Use a cold-water diffuser. Add the essential oils, one at a time directly on top of each other, in the water. You may also create a synergy. Add the oils to a clean dropper bottle, swirl to blend, and allow to synergize for 24 hours. Once synergized, add 4-12 drops to your diffuser.

NOTE: You may convert this recipe to a 5mL rollerball for a personal fragrance. Double or triple the recipe to your liking and combine all essential oils into a 5mL rollerball bottle, swirl to blend, and let synergize for 24 hours before topping off with V-6™ or Fractionated Coconut carrier oil. Apply on wrists and along sides of neck.

Grateful

Supports: Home air freshener and personal fragrance for feelings of emotional gratitude and thankfulness

Type: Cold-water Diffuser Blend

Ingredients:
- 3 drops Abundance™
- 3 drops Orange

Directions: Use a cold-water diffuser. Add the essential oils, one at a time directly on top of each other, in the water. You may also create a synergy. Add the oils to a clean dropper bottle, swirl to blend, and allow to synergize for 24 hours. Once synergized, add 4-12 drops to your diffuser.

NOTE: You may convert this recipe to a 5mL rollerball for a personal fragrance. Double or triple the recipe to your liking and combine all essential oils into a 5mL rollerball bottle, swirl to blend, and let synergize for 24 hours before topping off with V-6™ or Fractionated Coconut carrier oil. Apply on wrists and along sides of neck.

123

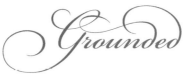

Grounded

Supports: Home air freshener and personal fragrance for feelings of emotional grounding and sense of calm

Type: Cold-water Diffuser Blend

Ingredients:
- 3 drops Northern Lights Black Spruce™
- 3 drops Frankincense
- 1 drop Geranium

Directions: Use a cold-water diffuser. Add the essential oils, one at a time directly on top of each other, in the water. You may also create a synergy. Add the oils to a clean dropper bottle, swirl to blend, and allow to synergize for 24 hours. Once synergized, add 4-12 drops to your diffuser.

NOTE: You may convert this recipe to a 5mL rollerball for a personal fragrance. Double or triple the recipe to your liking and combine all essential oils into a 5mL rollerball bottle, swirl to blend, and let synergize for 24 hours before topping off with V-6™ or Fractionated Coconut carrier oil. Apply on wrists and along sides of neck.

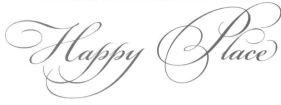

Supports: Home air freshener and personal fragrance for feelings of emotional happiness

Type: Cold-water Diffuser Blend

Ingredients:
- 2 drops Grapefruit
- 2 drops Lemon
- 2 drops Lime
- 2 drops Orange

Directions: Use a cold-water diffuser. Add the essential oils, one at a time directly on top of each other, in the water. You may also create a synergy. Add the oils to a clean dropper bottle, swirl to blend, and allow to synergize for 24 hours. Once synergized, add 4-12 drops to your diffuser.

NOTE: You may convert this recipe to a 5mL rollerball for a personal fragrance. Double or triple the recipe to your liking and combine all essential oils into a 5mL rollerball bottle, swirl to blend, and let synergize for 24 hours before topping off with V-6™ or Fractionated Coconut carrier oil. Apply on wrists and along sides of neck.

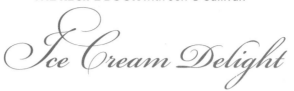

Ice Cream Delight

Supports: Home air freshener and personal fragrance for feelings of youth and delightful happiness

Type: Cold-water Diffuser Blend

Ingredients:
- 6 drops Tangerine
- 4 drops Lemon
- 1 drop Vanilla absolute

Directions: Use a cold-water diffuser. Add the essential oils, one at a time directly on top of each other, in the water. You may also create a synergy. Add the oils to a clean dropper bottle, swirl to blend, and allow to synergize for 24 hours. Once synergized, add 4-12 drops to your diffuser.

NOTE: Vanilla absolute may be purchased online at most herbal companies and is not the same as vanilla extract. You may convert this recipe to a 5mL rollerball for a personal fragrance. Double or triple the recipe to your liking and combine all essential oils into a 5mL rollerball bottle, swirl to blend, and let synergize for 24 hours before topping off with V-6™ or Fractionated Coconut carrier oil. Apply on wrists and along sides of neck.

Inspire

Supports: Home air freshener and personal fragrance for feelings of emotional inspiration and action

Type: Cold-water Diffuser Blend

Ingredients:

Recipe #1:
- 4 drops Motivation™
- 3 drops Frankincense
- 3 drops Jade Lemon

Recipe #2:
- 3 drops Inspiration™
- 3 drops Bergamot
- 2 drops Hinoki

Directions: Use a cold-water diffuser. Add the essential oils, one at a time directly on top of each other, in the water. You may also create a synergy. Add the oils to a clean dropper bottle, swirl to blend, and allow to synergize for 24 hours. Once synergized, add 4-12 drops to your diffuser.

NOTE: You may convert this recipe to a 5mL rollerball for a personal fragrance. Double or triple the recipe to your liking and combine all essential oils into a 5mL rollerball bottle, swirl to blend, and let synergize for 24 hours before topping off with V-6™ or Fractionated Coconut carrier oil. Apply on wrists and along sides of neck.

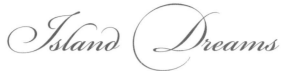

Island Dreams

Supports: Home air freshener and personal fragrance for feelings of open relaxation

Type: Cold-water Diffuser Blend

Ingredients:
- 3 drops Sandalwood
- 3 drops Orange

Directions: Use a cold-water diffuser. Add the essential oils, one at a time directly on top of each other, in the water. You may also create a synergy. Add the oils to a clean dropper bottle, swirl to blend, and allow to synergize for 24 hours. Once synergized, add 4-12 drops to your diffuser.

NOTE: You may convert this recipe to a 5mL rollerball for a personal fragrance. Double or triple the recipe to your liking and combine all essential oils into a 5mL rollerball bottle, swirl to blend, and let synergize for 24 hours before topping off with V-6™ or Fractionated Coconut carrier oil. Apply on wrists and along sides of neck.

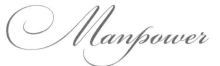

Manpower

Supports: Home air freshener and personal fragrance for feelings of emotional masculinity

Type: Cold-water Diffuser Blend

Ingredients:
- 3 drops Royal Hawaiian Sandalwood™
- 2 drops Tangerine
- 1 drop Cinnamon Bark
- 1 drop Vetiver

Directions: Use a cold-water diffuser. Add the essential oils, one at a time directly on top of each other, in the water. You may also create a synergy. Add the oils to a clean dropper bottle, swirl to blend, and allow to synergize for 24 hours. Once synergized, add 4-12 drops to your diffuser.

NOTE: You may convert this recipe to a 5mL rollerball for a personal fragrance. Double or triple the recipe to your liking and combine all essential oils into a 5mL rollerball bottle, swirl to blend, and let synergize for 24 hours before topping off with V-6™ or Fractionated Coconut carrier oil. Apply on wrists and along sides of neck.

Peace

Supports: Home air freshener and personal fragrance for feelings of emotional stability and peace

Type: Cold-water Diffuser Blend

Ingredients:
- 4 drops Patchouli
- 3 drops Tangerine
- 2 drops Orange

Directions: Use a cold-water diffuser. Add the essential oils, one at a time directly on top of each other, in the water. You may also create a synergy. Add the oils to a clean dropper bottle, swirl to blend, and allow to synergize for 24 hours. Once synergized, add 4-12 drops to your diffuser.

NOTE: You may convert this recipe to a 5mL rollerball for a personal fragrance. Double or triple the recipe to your liking and combine all essential oils into a 5mL rollerball bottle, swirl to blend, and let synergize for 24 hours before topping off with V-6™ or Fractionated Coconut carrier oil. Apply on wrists and along sides of neck.

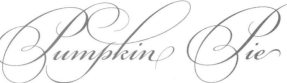
Pumpkin Pie

Supports: Home air freshener and personal fragrance for feelings of cozy family joy

Type: Cold-water Diffuser Blend

Ingredients:
- 3 drops Orange
- 2 drops Cinnamon Bark
- 2 drops Clove
- 2 drops Nutmeg
- 1 drop Ginger

Directions: Use a cold-water diffuser. Add the essential oils, one at a time directly on top of each other, in the water. You may also create a synergy. Add the oils to a clean dropper bottle, swirl to blend, and allow to synergize for 24 hours. Once synergized, add 4-12 drops to your diffuser.

NOTE: You may convert this recipe to a 5mL rollerball for a personal fragrance. Double or triple the recipe to your liking and combine all essential oils into a 5mL rollerball bottle, swirl to blend, and let synergize for 24 hours before topping off with V-6™ or Fractionated Coconut carrier oil. Apply on wrists and along sides of neck.

Romantical Nights

Supports: Home air freshener and personal fragrance for feelings of sensual openness

Type: Cold-water Diffuser Blend

Ingredients:
- 3 drops Grapefruit
- 2 drops Black Pepper
- 1 drop Jasmine

Directions: Use a cold-water diffuser. Add the essential oils, one at a time directly on top of each other, in the water. You may also create a synergy. Add the oils to a clean dropper bottle, swirl to blend, and allow to synergize for 24 hours. Once synergized, add 4-12 drops to your diffuser.

NOTE: You may convert this recipe to a 5mL rollerball for a personal fragrance. Double or triple the recipe to your liking and combine all essential oils into a 5mL rollerball bottle, swirl to blend, and let synergize for 24 hours before topping off with V-6™ or Fractionated Coconut carrier oil. Apply on wrists and along inner thighs.

132

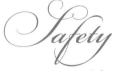

Safety

Supports: Home air freshener and personal fragrance for feelings of safety

Type: Cold-water Diffuser Blend

Ingredients:

Recipe #1:
- 4 drops Sacred Sandalwood™
- 4 drops Myrrh
- 2 drops Palo Santo

Recipe #2:
- 6 drops Christmas Spirit™
- 4 drops Bergamot
- 2 drops Cypress

Directions: Use a cold-water diffuser. Add the essential oils, one at a time directly on top of each other, in the water. You may also create a synergy. Add the oils to a clean dropper bottle, swirl to blend, and allow to synergize for 24 hours. Once synergized, add 4-12 drops to your diffuser.

NOTE: You may convert this recipe to a 5mL rollerball for a personal fragrance. Double or triple the recipe to your liking and combine all essential oils into a 5mL rollerball bottle, swirl to blend, and let synergize for 24 hours before topping off with V-6™ or Fractionated Coconut carrier oil. Apply on wrists and back of neck.

Seashore Breeze

Supports: Home air freshener and personal fragrance for feelings of calming bliss

Type: Cold-water Diffuser Blend

Ingredients:
- 5 drops Bergamot
- 4 drops Sandalwood
- 3 drops Grapefruit
- 1 drop Jasmine

Directions: Use a cold-water diffuser. Add the essential oils, one at a time directly on top of each other, in the water. You may also create a synergy. Add the oils to a clean dropper bottle, swirl to blend, and allow to synergize for 24 hours. Once synergized, add 4-12 drops to your diffuser.

NOTE: You may convert this recipe to a 5mL rollerball for a personal fragrance. Double or triple the recipe to your liking and combine all essential oils into a 5mL rollerball bottle, swirl to blend, and let synergize for 24 hours before topping off with V-6™ or Fractionated Coconut carrier oil. Apply on wrists and along back of neck.

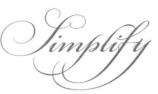

Simplify

Supports: Home air freshener and personal fragrance for feelings of simplicity

Type: Cold-water Diffuser Blend

Ingredients:
- 6 drops Lemon
- 3 drops Juniper
- 2 drops Geranium

Directions: Use a cold-water diffuser. Add the essential oils, one at a time directly on top of each other, in the water. You may also create a synergy. Add the oils to a clean dropper bottle, swirl to blend, and allow to synergize for 24 hours. Once synergized, add 4-12 drops to your diffuser.

NOTE: You may convert this recipe to a 5mL rollerball for a personal fragrance. Double or triple the recipe to your liking and combine all essential oils into a 5mL rollerball bottle, swirl to blend, and let synergize for 24 hours before topping off with V-6™ or Fractionated Coconut carrier oil. Apply on wrists and along back of neck.

135

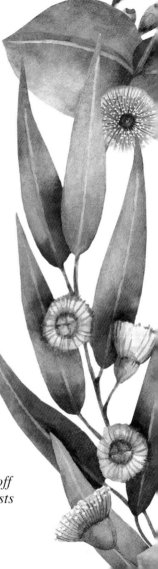

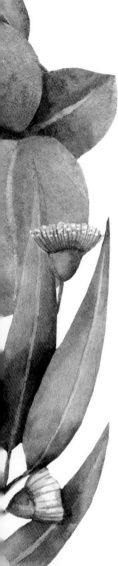

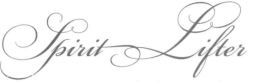

Spirit Lifter

Supports: Home air freshener and personal fragrance for uplifting spirits

Type: Cold-water Diffuser Blend

Ingredients:

Recipe #1:
- 4 drops Lavender
- 4 drops Orange
- 4 drops Spearmint

Recipe #2:
- 4 drops Tangerine
- 2 drops Joy®
- 1 drop Peppermint

Directions: Use a cold-water diffuser. Add the essential oils, one at a time directly on top of each other, in the water. You may also create a synergy. Add the oils to a clean dropper bottle, swirl to blend, and allow to synergize for 24 hours. Once synergized, add 4-12 drops to your diffuser.

NOTE: You may convert this recipe to a 5mL rollerball for a personal fragrance. Double or triple the recipe to your liking and combine all essential oils into a 5mL rollerball bottle, swirl to blend, and let synergize for 24 hours before topping off with V-6™ or Fractionated Coconut carrier oil. Apply on wrists and over heart area.

136

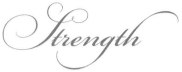

Strength

Supports: Home air freshener and personal fragrance for feelings of confidence and strength

Type: Cold-water Diffuser Blend

Ingredients:
- 5 drops Northern Lights Black Spruce™
- 2 drops Frankincense
- 2 drops Pine
- 2 drops Cedarwood
- 2 drops Bergamot

Directions: Use a cold-water diffuser. Add the essential oils, one at a time directly on top of each other, in the water. You may also create a synergy. Add the oils to a clean dropper bottle, swirl to blend, and allow to synergize for 24 hours. Once synergized, add 4-12 drops to your diffuser.

NOTE: Vanilla absolute may be purchased online at most herbal companies and is not the same as vanilla extract. You may convert this recipe to a 5mL rollerball for a personal fragrance. Double or triple the recipe to your liking and combine all essential oils into a 5mL rollerball bottle, swirl to blend, and let synergize for 24 hours before topping off with V-6™ or Fractionated Coconut carrier oil. Apply on wrists and along sides of neck and across forehead.

Uplift

Supports: Home air freshener and personal fragrance for feelings of emotional uplifting

Type: Cold-water Diffuser Blend

Ingredients:

Recipe #1:
- 6 drops Australian Kuranya™
- 2 drops Lemon
- 2 drops Grapefruit

Recipe #2:
- 4 drops Joy®
- 2 drops Myrrh
- 2 drops Orange

Directions: Use a cold-water diffuser. Add the essential oils, one at a time directly on top of each other, in the water. You may also create a synergy. Add the oils to a clean dropper bottle, swirl to blend, and allow to synergize for 24 hours. Once synergized, add 4-12 drops to your diffuser.

NOTE: Vanilla absolute may be purchased online at most herbal companies and is not the same as vanilla extract. You may convert this recipe to a 5mL rollerball for a personal fragrance. Double or triple the recipe to your liking and combine all essential oils into a 5mL rollerball bottle, swirl to blend, and let synergize for 24 hours before topping off with V-6™ or Fractionated Coconut carrier oil. Apply on wrists and along sides of neck.

138

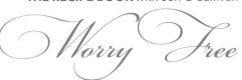

Worry Free

Supports: Home air freshener and personal fragrance for feelings of freedom from worry

Type: Cold-water Diffuser Blend

Ingredients:
- 6 drops Lime
- 3 drops Lavender
- 3 drops Cedarwood
- 2 drops Vanilla absolute

Directions: Use a cold-water diffuser. Add the essential oils, one at a time directly on top of each other, in the water. You may also create a synergy. Add the oils to a clean dropper bottle, swirl to blend, and allow to synergize for 24 hours. Once synergized, add 4-12 drops to your diffuser.

NOTE: Vanilla absolute may be purchased online at most herbal companies and is not the same as vanilla extract. You may convert this recipe to a 5mL rollerball for a personal fragrance. Double or triple the recipe to your liking and combine all essential oils into a 5mL rollerball bottle, swirl to blend, and let synergize for 24 hours before topping off with V-6™ or Fractionated Coconut carrier oil. Apply on wrists and along sides of neck.

139

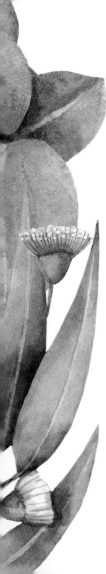

JADE LEMON™ & LEMON MYRTLE

Can you substitute Lemon Myrtle for Jade Lemon™? The short answer - no. Just because the word "lemon" is in the title does not necessarily mean it is from lemons. Lemon Myrtle (*Backhousia citriodora*) is from the Myrtaceae family and is steam distilled from the leaves of myrtle trees in Austrailia and is very similar in aroma to Lemon Verbena (*Aloysia citrodora*). Jade Lemon™ (*Citrus limon Eureka var. formosensis*) is from the Rutaceae family and is cold pressed from the rinds of lemons from Taiwan, China. A better substitute for Jade Lemon™ would be Lemon (*Citrus limon*). A better substitute for Lemon Myrtle would not be Myrtle (*Myrtus communis*) as you may suspect, but it would be Lemongrass (*Cymbopogon flexuosus*) as their constituents are most similar in therapeutic action. Below are the primary aromatic components of each oil.

JADE LEMON™ (EODR)
Rutaceae Family
Monoterpenes (70-90%):
• limonene (59-73%)
• β-pinene (7-16%)
• γ-terpinene (6-12%)
• α-pinene (1.5-3%)
• sabinene (1.5-3%)
Aldehydes (4-12%)
• citral (1-3%)
• citronellal (1-2%)
• geranial (1-2%)
• neral (1-2%)
• Plus others below 2%

LEMON (Average EODR & Online)
Ruraceae Family
Monoterpenes (70-90%):
• limonine (55-75%)
• β-pinene (7-16%)
• γ-terpinene (6-14%)
• α-pinene (1-3%)
• sabinene (1.5-3%)
Aldehydes (4-12%)
• citral (1-3%)
• citronellal (1-2%)
• geranial (1-2%)
• neral (1-2%)
• Plus others below 2%

LEMON MYRTLE
Myrtaceae family
• geranial (46-60%)
• neral (32-45%)
• Plus others below 4%

LEMONGRASS (*Cymbopogon flexuosus*)
Poaceae family
• geranial (32-47%)
• neral (22-38%)
• geraniol (5-10%)
• gernayl acetate (5-6%)
• Plus others below 5%

INFUSED BEVERAGE

Recipes

Infused Beer

Type: Infused Beverage

Ingredients:
- Recipe #1 Corona® Beer: Lime Vitality™
- Recipe #2 IPA Beer: Grapefruit Vitality™
- Recipe #3 Blue Moon® Beer: Orange Vitality ™
- Recipe #4 Stout Beer: Ginger Vitality ™

Directions: Add a drop of essential oil to empty glass first. Pour beer into the glass (do not use plastic cups or metal can). You may also drip one drop into a glass beer bottle and swirl before each sip.

Infused Champagne

Type: Infused Beverage

Ingredients:
Choose one of the following:
- 1 toothpick infused with Orange Vitality™
- 1 toothpick infused with Citrus Fresh Vitality™
- 1 toothpick infused with Grapefruit Vitality™
- 1 toothpick infused with Spearmint Vitality™
- 1 toothpick infused with Lime and Lavender Vitality™
- 1 toothpick infused with Jade Lemon Vitality™
- 1 toothpick infused with Bergamot Vitality™

Directions: Pour Champagne into a glass (do not use plastic). Dip a toothpick into the desired essential oil bottle, coating the toothpick half way. Tap off excess, and swirl into glass. Add a weight to the toothpick, such as a strawberry or lemon slice, to anchor the toothpick for continued flavor.

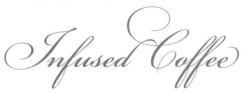

Infused Coffee

Type: Infused Beverage

Ingredients: (use only Young Living Vitality™ essential oils)
- Recipe #1 Dandy™ Blend: Thieves®
- Recipe #2 Regular Brew: Tangerine
- Recipe #3 Dark Roast: Cinnamon Bark
- Recipe #4 Light Roast: Ginger
- Recipe #5: Espresso: Clove
- Recipe #6 Cappuccino: Lavender
- Recipe #7 Latte: Peppermint
- Recipe #8 Mocha: Nutmeg

Directions: Dip a toothpick into the desired essential oil, tap off excess, and swirl into your cup of Dandy™ Blend or coffee. Add cream and sugar or honey as desired. Leave toothpick in cup for continued flavor. For bolder flavor, add one full drop to mug. Use metal spoon to stir before each sip. Feel free to mix and match any of the above combinations to your liking. Try adding a citrus Vitality™ essential oil to the combo.

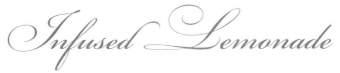

Type: Infused Beverage

Ingredients: (use only Young Living Vitality™ essential oils)
- Recipe #1: 1-2 drops Lavender
- Recipe #2: 3 drops Lime and 2 drops Peppermint
- Recipe #3: 2 drops Grapefruit and 2 drops Orange
- Recipe #4: 3 drops Citrus Fresh™
- Recipe #5: 1 drop Nutmeg and 1 drop Ginger
- Recipe #6: 1 drop Ginger and 2 drops Lemon
- Recipe #7: 2 drops Lavender and 1 drop Thyme
- Recipe #8: 2 drops each Grapefruit, Lime, and Tangerine

Directions: Make lemonade using 2 cups organic cane sugar, 8 cups water, and 2 cups fresh squeezed lemon juice. In a saucepan, combine sugar and 1 cup of water. Bring it to a boil, stirring continually until it is fully dissolved into a syrup. Allow syrup to cool to room temperature, then cover and place into refrigerator until chilled. Combine all ingredients into a pitcher (syrup, lemon juice, and additional 7 cups of water.) Add essential oils from one of the above recipes. Stir to blend well before pouring into a glass. Use stainless steel straws to sip from.

Infused NingXia Red®

Type: Infused Beverage

Ingredients:

Recipe #1:
- 1 drop Thieves Vitality™
- 2 drops Lemon Vitality™

Recipe #2:
- 1 drop Peppermint Vitality™
- 1 drop Orange Vitality™
- 1 drop Lemon Vitality™

Recipe #3:
- 3 drops Red Shot™
- 1 packet NingXia Nitro®

Recipe #4:
- 1 drop Lavender Vitality™
- 1 drop Lemon Vitality™
- 1 drop Peppermint Vitality™

Recipe #5:
- 1 drop Red Shot™
- 1 drop Grapefruit Vitality™
- 1 drop Nutmeg Vitality™

Recipe #6:
- 1 drop Cinnamon Bark Vitality™
- 2 drops Tangerine Vitality™

Directions: Put essential oils into a wine glass. Add 1-2 ounces of NingXia Red® and swirl to mix. Drink all at once.

Infused Shakes

Type: Infused Beverage

Ingredients: (use only Young Living Vitality™ essential oils)
Chocolate Recipes:

- Recipe #1: 1 drop Tangerine and 1 drop Peppermint
- Recipe #2: 1 drop Tangerine and 1 drop Cinnamon Bark
- Recipe #3: 1 drop Peppermint and 1 drop Lemon
- Recipe #4: 1 drop Nutmeg
- Recipe #5: 1 drop Peppermint

Vanilla Recipes:

- Recipe #6: 1 drop Lemon and 1 drop Grapefruit
- Recipe #7: 1 drop Cinnamon Bark
- Recipe #8: 1 drop Nutmeg and 1 drop Cinnamon Bark
- Recipe #9: 1 drop Thieves® and 1 drop Lemon
- Recipe #10: 1 drop Orange and 1 drop Tangerine

Directions: Using one of the Young Living® shake mixes, blend as you normally would, then add one of the above recipes to the shake and blend well.

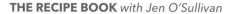

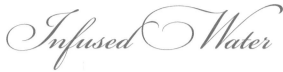

Type: Infused Beverage

Ingredients: (use only Young Living Vitality™ essential oils)
- Recipe #1: 2 drops Tangerine and 1 drop Peppermint
- Recipe #2: 2 drops Jade Lemon and 1 drop Spearmint
- Recipe #3: 1 drop each Orange and Grapefruit
- Recipe #4: 1 drop each Lime and Citrus Fresh™
- Recipe #5: 1 drop each Nutmeg and Cinnamon Bark
- Recipe #6: 2 drops Lime and 1 drop Lavender
- Recipe #7: 2 drops Lemon and 1 drop Peppermint
- Recipe #8: 2 drops Tangerine and 1 drop Ginger
- Recipe #9: 2 drops Orange and 1 drop Nutmeg
- Recipe #10: 1 drop each Lime, Grapefruit, and Lemon

Directions: Using a glass or stainless steel water bottle, add the essential oils from the desired recipe to the bottle, put a small dash of ground Pink Himalayan Salt into the bottle. Be careful not to add too much as you don't want your water to taste salty. Allow the essential oils to soak into the salt. Add cold water and swirl. Swirl bottle before each drink.

Infused Wine

Type: Infused Beverage

Ingredients:
- Recipe #1 Chardonnay: Tangerine Vitality™
- Recipe #2 Pinot Grigio: Jade Lemon Vitality™
- Recipe #3 Rosé: Grapefruit Vitality™
- Recipe #4 Pinot Noir: Citrus Fresh Vitality™
- Recipe #5 Cabernet Sauvignon: Cinnamon Bark Vitality™
- Recipe #6 Merlot: Orange Vitality™
- Recipe #7 Syrah: Nutmeg Vitality™

Directions: Pour wine into a glass (do not use plastic cups). Dip a toothpick into the desired essential oil, tap off excess, and swirl into the wine. Leave toothpick in glass for continued flavor. For bolder flavor, add one full drop to glass. Swirl glass before each sip.

Infused Chocolate

Type: Infused Dessert

Ingredients:
- Peppermint Vitality™
- Orange Vitality™
- Melting Chocolate
- Nuts, coconut, or powdered sugar (optional)
- Rice Krispies Treats®

Directions: Make a full sheet of Rice Krispies Treats® and pat down to be 1 inch deep in the pan. Cut into long "stick" pieces that are 1x1x2 or 1x1x3 inches. Put to the side. Melt chocolate and then add 1 drop Peppermint Vitality™ and 1 drop Orange Vitality™ and stir into mix. Put chopped nuts, coconut, or powdered sugar into a small bowl. Dip one end of each Rice Krispies Treat® into the chocolate, coating 1/4 to 1/2 the stick. Sprinkle desired topping onto the chocolate. Then stand upright on the rice paper like a tower, with the chocolate on the bottom. Place in refrigerator to set completely. Remove from refrigerator 30 minutes before consuming.

One Hundred Gifts

Type: BONUS Premium Starter Kit Gift Guide

Ingredients & Directions:
- See www.31oils.com/100gifts
- Samples on page 152

This bonus gift guide contains instructions on how to use your Premium Starter Kit with Young Living® to make 100 gifts. The recipes, supply lists, and even links to my favorite containers, base lotions, and other ingredients can be found at www.31oils.com/100gifts along with beautiful free printable labels.

Take a photo of your items and tag them on social media as #myEOcreation so we can all enjoy the fun and magic of making these easy and effective gifts!

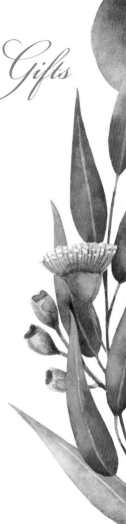

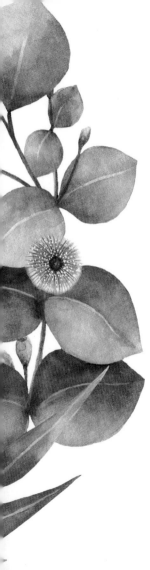

ONE HUNDRED GIFTS SAMPLE

Make 100 gifts using the Young Living™ Premium Starter Kit! Below are the items you will make and you may find the recipes along with the supplies needed at www.31oils.com/100gifts.

- Bath Salt: Makes 10 jars using 3 drops each Citrus Fresh™

- Candy Cane Hand Lotion & Hand Wash: Makes 10 sets using 2 drops each Peppermint and Lemon

- Holiday Bath Body Lotion & Body Wash Set: Makes 10 sets using 2 drops each Stress Away™

- Holiday Honey: Makes 10 jars using 3 drops Thieves®

- Just Breathe Rollers: Makes 10 rollers using 5 drops each Raven™

- Clarity Roller: Makes 10 rollers using 5 drops each PanAway®

- Mini Deluxe Eye Serum: Makes 10 serums using 2 drops each Lavender, Frankincense, Copaiba

- Candy Cane Cocoa: Makes 10 jars using 3 drops each Peppermint

- Holiday Herbal Drink: Makes 10 jars using 3 drops Thieves®

- Bathroom Toilet Air Freshener: Makes 10 spray bottles using Thieves® Cleaner Packet

FINAL THOUGHTS

Essential oils have become an integral and necessary part of my family's wellness practice. Creating recipes has become second nature. While people know me online for teaching with a shoot-from-the-hip style, the reason they come back is because the recipes I give them work. God has granted me the ability to understand notes and aromas, along with the finer details of synergistic therapeutic action. Synergizing specific essential oils is an art form, and I feel honored and blessed that God would allow me the ability to develop them and share them with you!

Being in the public eye has taught me one major thing: Give them what they want! You are my tribe and what my tribe always wants most is more recipes. As you move through this book, remember to jot down notes and star the recipes you love. Start to play a bit by modifying some that I have formulated to see if they work a little different. Also remember that if you don't have a specific oil, try to get it or simply leave it out. The main oils in each recipe are at the very top or closer to the top, so if an oil is listed at the bottom of the recipe and you do not have it, then simply leave it out. Very few essential oils can be substituted as their individual properties are specific and detailed.

A prime example would be with Sacred Frankincense™ (*Boswellia sacra*) and Frankincense (*Boswellia carterii*). Many people think one may be substituted for the other, but they have completely different constituents. See Lesson #12 in my book, "VITALITY, The Young Living Lifestyle." The same is true for Elemi and Frankincense.

A recent recommended substitution, that I am positive was an oversight, is the substituting of Lemon Myrtle for Jade Lemon. Just because the word "lemon" is in the title does not necessarily mean it is from lemons. Lemon Myrtle is steam distilled from the leaves of myrtle trees. Jade Lemon is cold pressed from the rinds of lemons from China. How these two got mixed up as similar is a mystery to me. If you do not have Jade Lemon, simply substitute it with Lemon. They are very similar, but still different.

Very few essential oils are close enough to be truly substituted. Two essential oils that come to mind that may be substituted is Sacred Sandalwood™ and Royal Hawaiian Sandalwood™. The constituents are very similar, but not the exact same. Read up on the title pages in this book about some of these differences between oils such as Angelica and White Angelica™, Melaleuca alternifolia (Tea Tree) and Melaleuca quinquernervia, along with Raven™, Ravensara, and Ravintsara.

Another common mistake is when a person does not have a particular essential oil, such as Rose, and they decide to substitute it with a blend that contains Rose, such as Joy®. That would be like using a cookie in your recipe that calls for butter simply because you are out of butter, and your cookie contains butter. The best method is to leave it out for now until you can purchase it. Or, better yet, find a friend that will lend you or sell you the necessary drops for your recipe... just like borrowing some eggs from your neighbor!

When you start to truly grasp the intricacies of each single species of essential oil, you will start to grasp the power behind them. They are phenomenal and are the reason formulating beautiful and powerful synergies and recipes can be so tremendously exciting! If you would like to try your hand at recipe development, the only thing stopping you is you. Start to play. Learn by smelling them, then feeling their action. I recommend getting the Vitality book so you can learn all about blending and notes. Your heart will sing as you find synergies that work just right specifically for your unique needs.

Thank you for enjoying this journey with me and I look forward to seeing you online. Don't forget to tag your Instagram recipes with the hashtag #myEOcreation so we can all learn together!

~ Jen O'Sullivan

ADDITIONAL EDUCATION

- Make 100 gifts using the Premium Starter Kit www.31oils.com/100gifts
- Supplies list at www.31oils.com/supplies
- Join the VITALITY Book Club for additional resources at www.Facebook.com/groups/VitalityBook
- Sign up for the eCourse at www.31oils.com/oils101
- Apps: "The EO Bar" and "Live Well with Young Living"
- Connect on Facebook: The Human Body and Essential Oils group
- Shareable Facebook Content: www.Facebook.com/JenOSullivanAuthor
- Instagram: @JenAuthor
- YouTube: www.JensTips.com
- Printed Resources: www.31oils.com
- Business Video Series: www.JenOSullivan.com

BOOKS BY JEN O'SULLIVAN

- VITALITY: The Young Living Lifestyle
- The Essential Oil Truth: The Facts Without the Hype
- French Aromatherapy: Essential Oil Recipes and Usage Guide
- Essentially Driven: Young Living Essential Oils Business Handbook
- Live Well (the PSK educational mini book)
- Essential Oil Make & Takes